# CONDUCTING HEALTH RESEARCH

## *with*

# NATIVE AMERICAN COMMUNITIES

*Edited by*
*Teshia G. Arambula Solomon, PhD,*
*and Leslie L. Randall, RN, MPH, BSN*

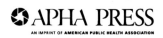

APHA PRESS
AN IMPRINT OF **AMERICAN PUBLIC HEALTH ASSOCIATION**

WASHINGTON, D.C. • 2014

American Public Health Association
800 I Street, NW
Washington, DC 20001-3710
www.apha.org

Georges C. Benjamin, MD, FACP, FACEP (Emeritus), Executive Director
Stephanie St. Pierre, MDiv, MPH, Publications Board Liaison

Printed and bound in the United States of America
*Book Production Editor:* Teena Lucas
*Typesetting:* The Charlesworth Group
*Cover Design:* Mazin Abdelgader
*Cover Art:* Gerald Cournoyer, *Across Two Worlds*
*Printing and Binding:* Sheridan Press Books, Inc.

Library of Congress Cataloging-in-Publication Data

Conducting health research with Native American communities / edited by Teshia G. Arambula Solomon, PhD, and Leslie L. Randall, RN, MPH, BSN.
        pages cm
    Includes bibliographical references and index.
    ISBN 978-0-87553-202-8
    1.   Indians of North America--Health and hygiene--Research. 2.   Alaska Natives--Health and hygiene--Research. 3.   Indigenous peoples--Health and hygiene--North America--Research. 4.   Pacific Islanders--Health and hygiene--Research. 5.   Public health--Research--North America. 6.   Health surveys--North America.
    7.   Health surveys--Islands of the Pacific.   I. Solomon, Teshia G. Arambula.   II. Randall, Leslie L.
    RA448.5.I5C66 2014
    362.1089'97--dc23

                                                                                                2013051062

# TABLE OF CONTENTS

# Dedication

Our journey to this book has been long. In the time period that we gave the first Continuing Education Institute to the present, life has rolled on for the authors. Some have moved homes (more than once), changed jobs (more than once), retired, earned doctorates, suffered illness, and lost loved ones. We would like to dedicate this book to:

- Those who have come before us and paved the road, that we may follow in their footsteps;
- Those who walk with us, and carry the burden of walking in two worlds to benefit our people;
- Those who will come after us, we hope to have eased your burden;
- Those we have lost, especially our co-author, colleague, and friend, Dr. Roxanne Struthers, who passed on December 10, 2005; may she smile upon us.

# Foreword

The current research and evaluation of the American Indian and Alaska Native (AIAN) people demonstrates the increased demand for efficiency, accompanied by solid accountability in a time of extremely limited resources. This environment requires proficiency in working with these vulnerable populations in diverse cross-cultural settings. Unfortunately, the available literature is lacking in providing adequate information to help researchers meet these demands. Thus, we welcome this timely publication.

The authors have a very solid and comprehensive understanding of work in this setting. They have special expertise developed over decades of working as researchers in AIAN communities, and have applied their knowledge by selecting key issues for discussion and examining the way in which these topics are applied to the AIAN community in a forthright manner. Essentially, the book provides an overview of complex themes as well as a synopsis of essential concepts or techniques in working with Native American tribes and Alaska Native communities. The benefits are to the Native people and organizations and to the researcher, whether a student just beginning research and evaluation activities, or an experienced practitioner, who may only need to refresh familiarity with topics and techniques not used on a regular basis.

Research and evaluation in Native American communities is important and needed. It is the only way to make rational choices between alternative practices, validate improvements, and build effective and safe practices to protect and improve the overall well-being and health of the people. It is critical to involve the people in the work, and not just as volunteer participants being studied–they should be involved as full partners in contributing to the design, execution, and analysis of the data obtained. This work touches on these important issues, and as a result, I know this will improve the quality of the literature.

I fully endorse this book as a timely contribution to building a stable foundation of effective practices of research and evaluation in Native American communities. When complemented by the sciences required to conduct good research and suggestions and comments from readers who have their own experiences from which to draw, it will help produce outcomes that have meaning and real application of advancing new knowledge in our dynamic and changing world. I believe it will benefit researchers and students of all levels of experience, tribal leaders, and Native community members. Finally, it provides critical and useful insights into the private and government agencies that approve research grants.

Phillip L. Smith, MD, MPH
Assistant Surgeon General, United States Public Health Service (retired)
Former Director of the Indian Health Service Planning
Evaluation and Research Program

# Acknowledgments

Bringing a book to life takes a great deal of time and great minds. The editors would like to thank each and every author, contributor, and the original speakers of the Continuing Education Institute (CEI):

Doris M. Cook, PhD, MPH
Francine C. Gachupin, PhD, MPH, CIP
Felicia Schanche Hodge, DrPH
Ben Muneta, MD, MPH
Leslie L. Randall, RN, MPH, BSN
Delight E. Satter, MPH
Phillip L. Smith, MD, MPH
Roxanne Struthers, RN, PhD, CHTP, AHN-BC, CTN
Lillian Tom-Orme, RN, PhD, MPH, FAAN

William L. Freeman, MD, MPH, CIP
Jennifer A. Giroux, MD, MPH
Jennie R. Joe, PhD, MPH
Joey Quenga, BA
Raynald Samoa, MD
Teshia G. Arambula Solomon, PhD
Maile Taualii, PhD, MPH
Thomas K. Welty, MD, MPH

Wendy Perry, MPA, senior analyst in the Office of the Director at the Agency for Healthcare Research Quality, encouraged us to put our thoughts on paper and supported us by providing advice and resources in order to disseminate this information widely. We offer our greatest gratitude to her.

We thank the American Public Health Association's (APHA's) editorial staff and board of directors for their patience and support for this project. The first editor we worked with at APHA was Ellen Meyer, now deceased. Ellen was an enthusiastic supporter of our little book. She always offered sage advice and understanding for novice editors. We miss her greatly, as she made the process joyful. Her replacement, Nina Tristani, also deserves a round of applause for picking up where we left off with Ellen, as do Teena Lucas, book production editor, and Robin Levin Richman, developmental editor, for seeing us through to the end. Multiple other staff members worked to bring this book to fruition and assisted in the online submission process. Stephanie St. Pierre in particular added invaluable insight into the development and editing of the chapters.

We thank the APHA for providing a platform from which to present our information both through the CEI and the books division. The American Indian, Alaska Native, and Native Hawaiian (AI/AN/NH) Caucus was established in 1981 to advocate for equal opportunity and access to quality health care for indigenous peoples of North America and the Hawaiian Islands. Through APHA, the AI/AN/NH Caucus promotes health policy to benefit Native populations.

Just as the AI/AN/NH Caucus provides a home for public health advocates to benefit Native communities, the Native Research Network, Inc. (NRN) provides a home for those interested in research by and for Native people. NRN is a network of Native researchers that promotes and advocates for high quality and principled research in Native communities. We are grateful to NRN for being supportive of this book and promoting its development through the years.

Drs. Robert S. Young and Jennie R. Joe have been our mentors and editors for longer than we wish to admit. We thank them for making us work hard to bring this book to fruition. We thank them and the rest of the team at the Native American Research and Training Center—Denise Angel, Christina Andrews, Carol Goldtooth Begay, Stacey Lopez, Ingrid Sam, and Jazmin Villavicencio—for their skilled literature searching and editing.

The cover artwork was generously provided by Lakota artist, Gerald Cournoyer (see http://www.geraldcournoyer.com). According to the artist, his painting *Across Two Worlds* depicts how Indian people are required to live in two worlds in order to become successful. We chose this painting as the cover for this book because it reflects the two worlds that those conducting research in native communities must walk in as well. We thank the artist for his generosity.

Last, we thank our Native people, families, and elders, for despite the many years of research, our overall health status remains the worst of any racial/ethnic subpopulation in the United States. We hope that our little book offers both an apology for all that has gone wrong and a blessing for moving forward in the future. For all that you have given us, we are forever grateful.

## SPECIAL ACKNOWLEDGMENT FROM THE NATIVE ISLANDER AUTHORS

The authors would like to extend their appreciation to the Pacific Islander community, for whom all of this is possible and intended to serve. We would also like to recognize that there are a number of key researchers in our community, many of whom have their own perceptions that may differ from those of the authors. The ideas and concepts in the book are intended to be a guide and not a prescription. Many years of research experience has allowed for these ideas to be developed and presented, and we are grateful to all of those who have come before us in service to the Pacific Islander people.

We would like to also recognize and honor our ancestors. As navigators of the largest body of water on the earth, they determined the course of new life and new investigation. As Pacific Islander researchers of today, we believe we are following the path laid out before us and we are humbled by its vision and breadth to serve all of our people.

*Mahalo Nui Loa, Si Yu'us Ma'ase, Fa'afetai Tele Lava, Yakoke, Qĕciyéẃyeẃ, Ahéhee', Miigwech, niawenko:wa, Masi, and Kaa, yeinyac (Thank you in Hawaiian, Chomorru, Samoan, Choctaw, Nez Perce, Dine', Ojibwe, Mohawk, Chinook wawa, and Wailiki)*

# Introduction
# The Essential Concepts: Core Values, Partnership, and Protection

Teshia G. Arambula Solomon, PhD, and
Leslie L. Randall, RN, MPH, BSN

Storytelling is at the core of who we are. It is the way we share information, make connections, find our relationships, learn, and teach. The stories we tell in this book are a reflection of all this, plus gratitude for the gifts we have been given: the opportunity to learn from our community, our partners. In this book we weave the voice of science—objective, distant, factual—and the voice of culture—subjective, close, experiential. We describe historical accounts and speak of our own experiences as Native investigators and the non-Natives who have made an effort to understand the culture and people. We walk in the space between contemporary science and Native tradition regularly in our work, so it is reasonable that we would also do this here. This is one of the greatest benefits of this book: we seek to create a relationship with the reader and weave together what we have learned from academia, our own traditions, and our personal experience as Native investigators.

## RATIONALE

The old saying "the road to hell is paved with good intentions" means that sometimes even when we intend to do good, things may not work out the way we plan. The histories of Indigenous people worldwide are littered with policies and practices of deliberate maltreatment, abuse, and criminal activity in the name of money, power, land, and religion, resulting in the all-too-common outcomes of poverty and poor health. Such acts are easy to condemn and criticize, and it is easy to understand why people are distrustful of government entities and other institutions and research in general.

Less obvious, however, are the problems created and the damage done when we try to be helpful. Presumably there are researchers and scientists who are unethical, fraudulent, and self-promoting, as there are such people in all walks of life. We have been fortunate because the majority of the people we have worked with are good people. They didn't go into health, science, or education to become rich or famous, but rather because of a desire to make a difference in the world, to be of service, and for the simple joy of learning and discovery. Unfortunately, even research done with good intentions has caused harm to individuals and communities.

Research is often something "done" to Native people without full disclosure by the researcher and full understanding and consent of these communities and individuals, rather than something conducted by them and for their benefit. It is not uncommon for researchers to come into a community, conduct a quick research project, and then leave, taking with them data, specimens, and community trust. Approvals to conduct the research are neither sought nor given, and if they are it is often without a complete understanding of purpose and benefit. The results and benefits are not shared, and permission to publish the results or any other information about the community are neither sought nor provided. The consequence of this approach is that Native people have a profound distrust of research, researchers, and the institutions that support them.

Many communities feel they have been over-researched and often there is little-to-no concrete evidence that the community of study has benefited from the research. For example, the Pima people of Arizona have been participants in diabetes research for over 50 years, providing valuable information for the development of pharmaceuticals like angiotensin-converting enzyme (ACE) inhibitors and angiotensin II (AT II) inhibitors to prevent end-stage renal disease. These discoveries have been a gold mine for pharmaceutical manufacturers; however, the death rates for Native American (NA) persons caused by diabetes are still astronomical, and little money or support has been returned to this community. In 1980, diabetes was the sixth leading cause of death among American Indians and Alaska Natives (AIANs), and in 2006 it was the fourth leading cause of death (CDC 2009). Death rates for the AIAN population (39.6/100,000) are nearly twice the rate of the Non-Hispanic White population (20.4/100,000; CDC 2010a) and for AIAN women, the disparity is even higher (40.7/100,000), nearly twice the rate of the Non-Hispanic White population (17.0/100,000; CDC 2010b). This old model of research is no longer welcome.

This book describes a philosophy and represents the current trend in Native communities of reclaiming power and sovereignty by controlling the research that is conducted in their name and on their lands. Although we only touch on tribal sovereignty and self-governance, there are many reference books and articles that address that issue in depth. Authors such as Deloria and Wilkins expound on the historical, cultural, and legal aspects, while authors such as Pevar and Canby cover the purely legal aspects of Indian law. We present here a model of the "how" with an appreciation of the "why." We offer a model that is collaborative and in which the community actively participates in the design, development, implementation, and evaluation of the research and benefit economically as well as regarding health outcomes. This philosophy embraces three essential concepts: (1) core values, (2) partnership, and (3) protection, which are intermingled within the larger context of culture.

All research should be consistent with the values of the population of study. Core values of Native communities such as family, respect, honesty, kindness, caring, and sharing should be honored. Research that uses conflicting methodologies may harm individuals and the community and offer no benefit to them. Throughout this book, the authors discuss common values across communities; this is particularly addressed in Joe's chapter on cultural competency. Cultural values are not always easily observed or expressed. Ignorance of these practices not only can lead to an unsuccessful research endeavor but also may lead to litigation or other ramifications, whereas being knowledgeable about them generally leads to success. The best way to be informed on culture, values, and traditions is to involve the communities of study in the research process. This is achieved through transparency and partnerships.

Throughout the book we use the term *participatory research*, which has come to be the model embraced by Native communities and is exemplified by the researchers who contributed to this book. A partnership between the researchers and the community should be brokered to the level desired by the community, encompassing all that the term legally and sociologically implies including sharing resources, profits, publication, and other forms of recognition. There should be transparency in all transactions and they should be negotiated with the community of study prior to submission of an application. Any benefits, financial or otherwise, must be shared equitably with the study population and the community. Those who have participated in the production of this book are known as researchers who have abided by the wishes of the community for years, have shared their knowledge of the research with the community, have been to the community to consult with and report back their findings, and are respected by the communities with whom they work, and the majority are Native themselves.

As a result of a history of abuse and neglect, Native communities must protect themselves through self-determination and self-governance. Indigenous knowledge must be protected as one protects those things that are sacred in the major religions, and intellectual property rights must remain with the elders or other knowledge holders within the community. Through the creation and implementation of respectful partnerships, cultural protocols and traditions will be inherently protected and respected. As with all research, individual consent is mandatory. But because Native people may have difficulty with language or reading or simply understanding the culture of research, we must go the extra distance to ensure that consent is truly fully informed. A full and informed consent from individuals and the community may require tactics such as video consent or translation when language and literacy are an issue. It is important to note that the legal language used by most research institutions is often confusing to the participants, and the institutional review board (IRB) forms that protect the research institution may not be sufficient to protect the individual or the community. Confidentiality is also a common protection afforded in health research; however, for Native communities in which populations are particularly small, this issue becomes imperative. Confidentiality, anonymity, and public recognition must be negotiated before presentations or publications are made public. Study participants or community leaders should be co-authors on presentations and publications and should have the opportunity to review and revise. Data sharing, management, and reporting should all be determined *a priori* and with shared control, with the understanding that most Native communities will assert sovereignty and ownership of all data and that the researchers may not keep copies of data for their own use.

This book grew out of presentations originally given in 2000 as a Continuing Education Institute (CEI) at the 129th Annual Meeting of the American Public Health Association (APHA). Since that time the editors and authors have experienced all that life has to offer, including multiple moves across the country with job changes, retirements, births, hardships, illness, losses, and deaths. We have, however, persevered and are delighted to bring this edition to fruition.

## ORGANIZATION

The first half of the book provides a foundational context within which research occurs. Chapter 1 is a brief overview of AIAN history and politics in the United States to give the reader a framework for understanding how history and politics have influenced Native communities and why they are so resistant to and distrustful of research. In Chapter 2 we examine the difficulty in measuring and describing health patterns in Native communities because of data limitations that cloak our problems. Once this foundation of understanding is built, Randall, in Chapter 3, draws upon her extensive career in NA health for an introduction to working with Native communities, the essence of which is relationship building, and highlights briefly various research guidelines developed in other Indigenous communities. Chapter 4 then stresses the importance of understanding the unique cultural foundation of distinct and individual tribal nations. In Chapter 5, Taualii, Quenga, and Samoa introduce the reader to common problems facing Native Hawaiians and Pacific Islanders.

The second half of the book presents examples of research projects in the form of case studies of specific experiences. Hodge and Struthers in Chapter 6 and Tom-Orme in Chapter 7 open our eyes to successful models and methods of working in Native communities, and in Chapter 8 Welty provides living examples. Chapter 9 provides the opposite side of the coin, that is, what happens when things do not go as intended.

Last, we provide guidance in the ethical conduct of research. In Chapter 10 Cook describes a model process for developing research policy, the keystone to ethical conduct, and Gachupin and Freeman in Chapter 11 review the specifics of research that utilizes biospecimens.

## TERMINOLOGY

Determining who is and is not a Native American is a complex issue, and different groups have different positions on how people are described. In general, most Native people want to be referred to by the tribe to which they belong; for example, the Choctaw Nation or the Nimiipuu (Nez Perce). However, we rarely speak about individual communities for all the reasons described in this book and instead usually refer to people in the aggregate. In this book we use the term *Native American* or *American Indian* to describe the Indigenous peoples of Canada, the contiguous United States, Alaska, the Hawaiian islands, and the islands of Guam and American Samoa. American Indians and Alaska Natives are part of 566 federally recognized and more than 100 state-recognized tribal nations (tribes, nations, bands, pueblos, communities, rancherias, and native villages) in the United States, approximately 229 of which are located in Alaska.

Some people use the terms *Indigenous* or *Indian* interchangeably for American Indians or Native Americans. However, *Indigenous* refers to the original peoples of a geographic area; for example, the Indigenous people of New Zealand are the Maori. The term may be used when referring collectively to original peoples of many lands. *Indian* can also be confused for reference to the people of India, but in this book, it's obvious that we are referencing American Indians. Some people may use the term *Indian country* to refer to all the tribal communities across the United States.

Indigenous islanders are often grouped together and termed Native Hawaiian and Other Pacific Islanders or grouped with the Asian population as the Asian/Pacific Islander population. As described in Chapter 5, the term *Native American Islanders* refers to descendants of the original Natives of Hawai'i, Guam, Samoa, or other Pacific Islands.

In Canada, there are three politically and culturally distinct groups that comprise the 1,172,790 Aboriginal peoples of Canada (about 3.3% of the Canadian population): (1) First Nations, (2) Inuit, and (3) Métis. Aboriginal peoples are both the fastest growing and youngest population in Canada, as they experienced a 45% increase in population growth between 1996 and 2006, compared with an 8% increase for the non-Aboriginal population (Statistics Canada 2008).

## SUMMARY

This book was designed for those with good intentions to understand the potential pitfalls and outcomes of even the most well-intentioned research projects. Conducting research in Indian country can be a truly rewarding experience. NA people are generally warm, welcoming, and generous, but conducting research in their communities can be truly challenging, as Native Americans are a proud people with a well-earned distrust of outsiders. Being a Native researcher is not a license to conduct research in any Native community. Even researchers with proven track records and in good standing among NA communities will run into obstacles with their projects. Approval processes can be long, tribal politics can be an impediment, and research sites can be distant.

We hope this book will benefit those who are unfamiliar with Indigenous community research, its history, and politics, particularly those who are responsible for collecting data on the health and well-being of Native people (including academic researchers and public health officials at all levels of government), and that it will serve as a guide and a model for conducting respectful research in all communities. It is our greatest hope that Native communities will benefit from this book, not only through the education of the uninformed but also in building the capacity within their own communities to create a dialogue surrounding the research enterprise, for Native people will only be truly protected when they develop the capacity to direct, fund, and implement their own research, following well-developed research agendas and training high-quality Native researchers.

We also offer a note of caution that simply reading a book does not make one an expert, nor does writing one. If we clearly communicate only one message it is that the researcher must have an intimate understanding of the beliefs, values, and practices of the community of study and must both know and understand the laws of that community before embarking on a course of research. The only way to do that is by investing time in building partnerships with the community government and its people. In fact, that single statement is a perfect example; just as the US government is distal to us as individual US citizens, so are our tribal governments. Having a relationship with one is not sufficient; you must also have a relationship with both the tribal government and the community it is elected to serve. While tribal governments can vet you and grant you entrée, it is individual Native people who consent to participate. We hope you enjoy the book and wish you the best of luck in joining us to serve our Native brothers and sisters.

## REFERENCES

Centers for Disease Control and Prevention. 2009. *National Vital Statistic Report. Vol. 56, Num 10 Table 17 and Table 16.* Available at: http://www.cdc.gov/nchs/data/nvsr/nvsr57/nvsr57_14.pdf. Accessed July 10, 2013.

Centers for Disease Control and Prevention. 2010a. *Health United States, 2009. Table 26.* Available at: http://www.cdc.gov/nchs/data/hus/hus09.pdf. Accessed July 10, 2013.

Centers for Disease Control and Prevention. 2010b. *Health, United States, 2009: In Brief–Medical Technology.* Available at: http://www.cdc.gov/nchs/data/hus/hus09_InBrief_MedicalTech.pdf. Accessed July 10, 2013.

Statistics Canada. 2008. *2006 Census, Aboriginal Peoples.* Available at: http://www12.statcan.gc.ca/census-recensement/2006/rt-td/ap-pa-eng.cfm. Accessed September 13, 2013.

# The Complexity of American Indian and Alaska Native Health and Health Research: Historical, Social, and Political Implications for Research

Delight E. Satter, MPH, Leslie L. Randall, RN, MPH, BSN, and Teshia G. Arambula Solomon, PhD

## INTRODUCTION

Understanding the historic and current social and political context in which tribes and American Indian and Alaska Native (AIAN) communities function will assist the researcher in communicating with and building strong relationships in AIAN country. A review is provided of the historic relations between American Indians and Alaska Natives and the US government as well as demographic information, key definitions, policies relevant to public health, and the research concerns of racial underreporting and misclassification specific to American Indians and Alaska Natives.

## A BRIEF HISTORY

The violence, trauma, and oppression experienced by American Indians and Alaska Natives over the past 500 years has created an aura of distrust of federal and state governments and their agents, healthcare providers, scientists, and researchers. Historical accounts show that tens of millions of Indigenous people, both in North and South America, died as a result of the European exploration of the New World (Verano and Ubelaker 1991). These deaths occurred primarily through the introduction of infectious diseases, slavery, and warfare (Bryan 1999). The spread of epidemic diseases such as smallpox, measles, whooping cough, bubonic plague, malaria, yellow fever, diphtheria, and influenza decimated up to 90% of the Indigenous population (Bryan 1999). The methods of introduction of some diseases into these communities by non-Native contacts were at times intentional and destructive. For example, smallpox was spread through the distribution of blankets infected with the disease specifically to eliminate tribal people in order to seize their lands (Verano and Ubelaker 1991). This history has deeply influenced interactions between tribal communities and all non-Indians, including researchers.

After the founding of the United States, through the passage of acts of Congress, governmental policies were established to eliminate or assimilate American Indians and Alaska Natives. Between 1830 and 1850, the Indian Removal Act forced the relocation of the majority of the eastern tribes to lands west of the Mississippi River, with a purpose of opening land occupied by tribes to non-Indian people; this practice continued into the 20th century (Getches et al. 2004, Deloria et al. 1983, Perdue and Green 1995). From 1850 to 1871, Congress implemented the reservation system as part of its policy to forcibly remove American Indians from their homelands. The creation of over 100 treaties either moved tribes to new territories or confined them to smaller territories. During the Assimilation and Allotment Era, from 1871 to 1928, the US government sold or gave Indian land to non-Indians in an attempt to assimilate Indians into US culture. This resulted in a loss of 90 million of the 138 million acres of Indian territory originally allotted from 1850 to 1871 and the displacement of thousands of Indians (Deloria and Wilkins 2000). In addition, children were targeted for removal to Indian boarding schools as a tactic to destroy the traditional cultural knowledge passed from generation to generation (Holt 2001). This was an effective strategy to eliminate cultural and familial ties. As stated in the Meriam Report (Brookings Institution 1928):

> The survey staff finds itself obliged to say frankly and unequivocally that the provisions for the care of the Indian children in boarding schools are grossly inadequate.

And:

> The discipline in the boarding schools is restrictive rather than developmental. Routine institutionalism is almost the invariable characteristic of the Indian boarding school.

And:

> Ultimately, most of the boarding schools as at present organized should disappear.

Under a more Indian-friendly federal government, Congress passed the Indian Reorganization Act of 1934, which reaffirmed tribal governments and recognized the sovereignty of the tribes. Unfortunately, the government policy of termination of Indian tribes between 1943 and 1968 ended treaty ties between Indian tribes and the US government, reversing many of the reforms and once again promoting assimilation of Indians. The cumulative effect of each government effort resulted in acculturation or assimilation of tribal members. As a result, many of the tribes targeted for termination and relocation to reservations suffered extensive trauma and loss, including loss of culture and identity, traditional healing practices, self-esteem, and social structure while experiencing an increase in alcohol and substance abuse, morbidity, and mortality (Wissow 2000, Nelson and Manson 2000).

In what some people considered another ambitious effort at solving the "Indian problem," a movement to sterilize without consent occurred from the 1970s through the early 1980s in parts of the Indian Health Service (IHS; the federal health program for American Indians and Alaska Natives). During this time, more liberal sterilization recommendations by the American College of Obstetricians and Gynecologists helped to increase sterilization rates in all populations in the United States (DeFine 1997). Sterilization was and is more common in non-White populations than in the White, non-Hispanic population (Mosher et al. 2004): for example, in 1982, 15% of White women, 24% of African-American women, 35% of Puerto Rican women, and 42% of AIAN women had been sterilized (DeFine 1997). During the 1970s, AIAN women reported coerced sterilization. In 1976 the Government Accounting Office (GAO) conducted a review of IHS records and concluded that there was uniformly a lack of informed consent from women undergoing sterilization and recommended improved consent procedures (Comptroller of the US

1976). In 1976, unconsented sterilization (hormonal and surgical) was still the most common method of birth control for all women in AIAN women; by 2002, oral contraceptive pills had become the most common method of birth control followed by surgical sterilization (Volscho 2009, Pinkerton-Uri 1974).

Investigations by Indian physicians and by Marie Sanchez, a tribal judge with the Northern Cheyenne, included interviews with women that illustrate the difference in value systems between AIAN women and the physicians "taking care" of them. The women were often told they had too many children and that they should stop having children, implying that the number of children they had was inappropriate (Dillingham 1977a, Dillingham 1977b, GAO 1976, Larson 1977). Awareness of the sterilization allegations and the documentation of other unconsented research created an atmosphere of distrust within tribal communities for non-Indians that continues to the present.

## TRIBAL SOVEREIGNTY

Most Americans perceive AIAN status solely as a racial minority issue (Kickingbird and Rhoades 2000). However, the status of tribal sovereignty of American Indians and Alaska Natives is secured by treaty with the US government, resulting in a government-to-government relationship similar to the relationship between the federal government and the states (Deloria and Lytle 1998). This status is reserved only for tribes recognized by the federal government under treaty or under a federal recognition process. A major misunderstanding of the treaty process is that sovereignty is "given" to tribes. Actually, Indian governments have inherent sovereignty, a status recognized by the United States (Kickingbird and Rhoades 2000).

Public Law 93–638, the Indian Self-Determination and Education Assistance Act of 1975 (ISDEA), is considered the single most important piece of legislation for American Indians. This law allows tribes to administer federal programs, including health services, within their tribal reservations. Tribes utilize either of two administrative mechanisms: the Title I process in which services are contracted through the IHS, or through the Title III process (self-governance), whereby tribes receive money directly from Congress. As stated on the IHS Web site:

As of December 2011, the IHS and Tribes have negotiated 82 self-governance compacts that are funded through 107 funding agreements with 337 (or nearly 60%) of the 566 federally recognized Tribes. This program constitutes approximately $1.5 billion (or 35 %) of the IHS budget. (IHS, Office of Tribal Self Governance)

However, the definition of self-determination varies by tribe. Some tribes believe that self-determination includes the treaty and trust obligation of the US government to provide healthcare, while others believe self-determination means assuming control over their own healthcare and making and enforcing their own laws including those governing research (Grim 2004).

In August 2000, President Clinton signed into law H.R. 1167, the Tribal Self-Governance Amendments of 2000, which amended the ISDEA by providing for further self-governance by Indian tribes. In June 2002, the Final Rule implementing Title V of the Tribal Self-Governance Amendments of 2000 (the Act) repealed Title III of the ISDEA and established a permanent self-governance program within the Department of Health and Human Services. Because of this law, tribes are now taking over their own healthcare, developing their own research agendas, and becoming more sophisticated about research.

## CONTRACTING, COMPACTING, AND IHS FUNDING STRUCTURE UNDER 638

What is a 638 contract and how is it different from compacting and IHS funding? A 638 contract is awarded to those tribes who wish to assume control over all or portions of their healthcare through a contracting process with IHS. It differs from compacting in that the money goes through IHS and is awarded as a contract to the tribe instead of directly from Congress. Some of the services that are contracted are alcohol treatment programs, community health representatives (CHRs), community health nursing (CHNs), and outpatient clinics (Dixon and Roubideux 2001).

What is compacting? According to the Tribal Self Governance Amendments of 2000, compacting is the transfer of "full control and funding to tribal governments, upon tribal request, over decision making for Federal programs, services, functions, and activities (or portions thereof)." (Tribal Self-Governance Amendments of 2000, P.L. 106-260, 114 Stat. 711 s2 [August 18, 2000]). This means that the funds necessary for operation of healthcare—

including any services that the tribe feels they can assume control over that were previously IHS functions—go directly to tribes from Congress rather than through the IHS, thus reducing the overall IHS budget. IHS then provides for the remainder of tribal services through hospitals, service units (made up of one or more ambulatory care units), health centers (clinics plus other preventive health services), and clinics (ambulatory care units) with funding provided directly from Congress to IHS. There are certain services that are considered essential to the functioning of IHS, and these are maintained at the area or national level (the United States is divided up into 12 regions with administrative offices called areas). Prior to compacting, the process was fairly simple. The money came from Congress to the IHS and from IHS to direct and contract services for the tribes or urban programs. Now, however, the system is more complex with a variety of compacted and contracted services across the nation and within an area or tribe.

## DEFINING AMERICAN INDIAN AND ALASKA NATIVE STATUS

Members of federally recognized tribes have legal rights to healthcare established by treaties, case law, the Snyder Act of 1921, the Indian Health Care Improvement Act, and the Tribal Self-Governance Amendments of 2000 (see earlier discussion). This legislation provides for government-to-government relationships between the United States and tribes. Grasping this concept is critical: it should be used as a touchstone for critically evaluating rights and responsibilities in conducting research with American Indians and Alaska Natives.

AIAN history makes defining who is a member of this political minority a complicated issue. Each tribe establishes its own criteria for tribal membership. Common criteria include a quarter tribal blood quantum level and evidence of descent from a tribal member or being recognized by other tribal members as belonging to the tribe. A tribe is any Indian tribe, band, nation, rancheria, pueblo, or other organized group or community, including any Alaska Native village, group, or regional or village corporation as defined in, or established by, the Alaska Native Claims Settlement Act (Kickingbird and Rhoades 2000), and as such, is recognized as eligible for the special programs and services provided by government-to-government entities to Indians through treaties. A tribe may be federally recognized, state recognized, or self-recognized. Federally recognized tribes have recognition and a unique relationship with the

US government (e.g. the Confederated Tribes of Grand Ronde, OR); state-recognized tribes do not have official recognition from the United States, but are recognized by their respective state governments (e.g. the Lumbee Tribe of North Carolina); and self-recognized tribes do not have recognition from the federal government or their home state but have historically held treaties with other nations (e.g. the Kawaiisu of California with Spain).

The term *Alaska Native* collectively refers to Eskimos, Aleuts, and American Indians who are indigenous to Alaska. The term *American Indian* includes enrolled members of federal or state recognized tribes as well as people who are self-identified as American Indian on the US Census and other similar reports. The terms *American Indian* and *Native American* technically refer to people having origins in North, Central, and South America, and who maintain tribal affiliation or community attachment. In this book, the term *American Indian and Alaska Native*, or *AIAN*, refers to descendants of tribes indigenous to what is now known as the United States. In no way does this definition serve to fundamentally exclude Indians indigenous to the Americas outside US borders. In reporting studies in tribes and Native communities, the most specific terminology allowed by the tribe should be utilized in order to provide the most accurate data and information.

A reservation is the geographic area reserved by treaty or other law for a federally recognized Indian tribe. Some reservations cross state lines and national borders. For example, the Navajo Nation includes parts of three contiguous states, and the Mohawk Nation of Akwesasne straddles the international boundaries of Canada and the United States, two Canadian provinces, and the New York State line. Contrary to popular belief, not all American Indians and Alaska Natives live on reservations. According to the US Census (2010), 71% of American Indians and Alaska Natives live in urban areas.

Tribes have varying governance systems, with either a government structured under the Indian Reorganization Act (IRA) of 1934 or a self-developed structure, with the primary difference being that IRA tribes have access to loans under the federal government, while non-IRA tribes (such as the Navajo) do not. As Pevar states: "Today, most tribal governments have the same three branches as the federal and state governments: legislative, executive and judicial" (1992). Most have adopted written constitutions but not all (e.g., the Navajo) and tribal codes. Some enforce their laws in their own courts;

others depend on federal agencies to maintain law and order on the reservation and allow states to have limited jurisdiction on most reservations unless the reservation is what is commonly referred to as a "checkerboard" reservation, meaning some of the land is non-Indian owned. In this instance, states and counties have jurisdiction unless a crime is committed by an Indian on Indian-owned or tribal land (Canby 1998, Pevar 1992, Wilkins and Lomawaima 2001). In their work, Wilkins and Lomawaima bring up an important point in state, federal, and tribal relationships:

> Aside from these few exceptions, states have no legitimate constitutional authority inside Indian Country, unless they obtain direct tribal and congressional invitation, an amendment of the state's statutory and constitutional laws, and arguably, a modification of existing Indian treaties.

This has been a cause of contention between states and tribes for years.

## INDIAN HEALTHCARE

Key policies throughout the 20th century have had an impact on the health and healthcare services of American Indians and Alaska Natives. The Snyder Act of 1921 was the first effort by Congress to improve general healthcare (Johnson and Rhoades 2000). The act sought to provide "relief of distress and conservation of health of Indians" but was consistently underfunded. In 1926, officers from the Commissioned Corps of the Public Health Service (PHS) were assigned to Indian health programs (Shelton 2001). In 1955 responsibility for delivering healthcare to American Indians and Alaska Natives transferred from the Interior Department's Bureau of Indian Affairs to IHS. For several decades, the government pursued a policy of assimilation and termination until 1968, when the Indian Civil Rights Act was passed, ending the unilateral extension of state jurisdiction over tribes and beginning the strengthening and restoration of tribal self-determination. Self-determination was made a reality when President Nixon, in his 1970 message to Congress, called for restoration and strengthening of tribal sovereignty and promotion of tribal self-governance. This became a legal reality when the ISDEA of 1975 and the Indian Health Care Improvement Act of 1976 was signed into law by President Ford. These two acts have had an inestimable effect on sovereignty for AIAN persons (Deloria 1984). The ISDEA was amended in 1992 to authorize a Self-Governance Demonstration Program in IHS to enable selected tribes to investigate self-determination for healthcare services. Further amendments resulted in H.R. 1167. This law allows all tribes to enter into the arena of administration of federal programs within their tribal reservations including, but not limited to, health services either through a Title I process whereby they may contract the services through IHS or through a Title V (which replaced Title III and established a permanent self-governance program) process whereby they may compact the services (Johnson and Rhoades 2000). An excerpt from the ISDEA shows the primary reasons for the law:

> The Congress, after careful review of the Federal Government's historical and special legal relationship with, and resulting responsibilities to, American Indian people, finds that
>
> (1) The prolonged Federal domination of Indian service programs has served to retard rather than enhance the progress of Indian people and their communities by depriving Indians of the full opportunity to develop leadership skills crucial to the realization of self-government, and has denied to the Indian people an effective voice in the planning and implementation of programs for the benefit of Indians which are responsive to the true needs of Indian communities; and
>
> (2) The Indian people will never surrender their desire to control their relationships both among themselves and with non-Indian governments, organizations, and persons.

Finally, the Indian Child Welfare Act of 1978 also provided for a range of human services, particularly social and mental health services (Shelton 2001). However, despite the attempts at reform, 35% of American Indians and Alaska Natives nationally report that they do not have a usual source of care, which is more than three times the proportion of those who have some form of health insurance coverage or who participate in the IHS system (Brown et al. 2002).

Uninsured American Indians and Alaska Natives are less likely to see a physician than other uninsured groups. Approximately half (49%) of American Indians and Alaska Natives younger than 65 years have job-based or private insurance as compared with 83% of the US White population of the same age (Zuckerman et al. 2004). However, American Indians and Alaska Natives who are covered by IHS only are more likely to identify a usual source of care, but are less likely to have the minimum number of doctor visits for their age group and health status (Brown et al. 2002). AIAN members who live on or near federal reservation lands receive universal healthcare at no charge through IHS. Basic healthcare is provided to all patients along with basic prescription needs at all times but when IHS or tribal healthcare funds run out before the end of the year, everyone is required to hold off on any outside contracted services until the following fiscal year (Dixon and Roubideaux 2000).

IHS's estimated service population for the year 2010 was 1.5 million (IHS 2011). Although more tribes have been successful in obtaining federal recognition, little or no increase in service dollars have been allocated to IHS to be inclusive of these communities (IHS 1999).

As mentioned, IHS provides primary care (along with hospital services) on-site; these services are primarily on remote reservations and available on a limited number of urban sites. IHS is limited in its sponsored services due to limited appropriations from Congress. AIAN persons eligible for services through IHS or urban Indian clinics are NOT excluded from participation in any other public insurance program, but individuals are often encouraged to access IHS clinics first rather than accessing other public services. Unfortunately, it is also IHS policy to advocate for use of alternate sources of health and healthcare funds first rather than IHS. Therefore, delays in accessing healthcare are often a result of disagreements among agencies regarding who is the appropriate payer (e.g., between Medicare and IHS; Dixon and Roubideaux 2000).

Tribal councils mandate who is eligible for healthcare within the federal guidelines for the funds they receive for their clinics. Most tribes require that a member must meet the following requirements:

(1)   be an enrolled tribal member or a descendant of a tribal member;
(2)   reside on the reservation or tribal territory or within 75 miles (some tribes are thinking of restricting this to 50 miles or less) for at least six months prior to requesting healthcare services; and
(3)   obtain their care at their home reservation tribal or IHS clinic.

As tribal member numbers increase and more American Indians and Alaska Natives move to areas where they cannot access their usual sources of healthcare, the restrictions are becoming more stringent. One reservation outside a major metropolitan area has recently begun restricting their services to those who live within the reservation; services are also limited for descendants. They had previously been providing services to individuals from the metropolitan area who could travel to the reservation to access their clinic (personal communication, NPAIHB Tribal Health Directors meeting, 2005). These can be major barriers to the majority of American Indians and Alaska Natives without eligibility or access to clinics and services (Kickingbird and Rhoades 2000).

The *Patient Protection and Affordable Care Act* (ACA) signed by President Obama on March 23, 2010, has implications for Native populations that are primarily positive. It enacted the Indian Health Care Improvement Act (IHCIA) as permanent for the first time since it was introduced in 1994 and amended each year until 2010. A challenge to the ACA was submitted to the Supreme Court that put IHCIA in question, but the final ruling in 2012 favored the act. The act also reauthorized programs for Native Hawaiians until 2019 (US Senate Committee on Indian Affairs 2010). As the ACA is implemented it is expected to impact several elements of the IHCIA: state-based health exchanges, no cost-sharing or co-payments, untaxable value of health services, Medicaid expansion, closing the Medicare "donut hole," and third-party reimbursements; further information regarding these elements can be found at http://www.nihb.org, http://www.ncai.org, and http://www. healthcare.gov. The ACA also expands IHS services including mental and behavioral health, increases clinician recruitment and retention in tribally operated health programs, and increases access to federal insurance. In the first months of 2013, the Centers for Medicare and Medicaid Services (CMS), the Department of Health and Human Services, and the Internal Revenue Service planned listening sessions with tribal leaders on the provisions for tribes and tribal members (Tribalhealthcare.org 2013). Time will tell how it will ultimately have an impact on Native populations within the United States.

## UNDERREPORTING AND MISCLASSIFICATION

The AIAN population is increasing at a rate of 1.8% a year, not including tribes newly gaining federal recognition. According to the 2010 US Census, 2.9 million US residents reported being solely of AIAN origin, with approximately 2.3 million additional residents reported being American

Indian or Alaska Native in combination with one or more other races. This is an increase of 40% from the 2000 US Census for those reporting AIAN status in combination with one or more other races and an 18% increase for those reporting AIAN status alone. California reported the greatest number of AIAN residents (627,600). Oklahoma reported the second highest number of AIAN residents (391,900). Life expectancy for AIAN persons for 2002 to 2004 was 72.5 years, compared with 77.5 years for all races and 78.0 years for Whites. The AIAN population is also younger than the US population for all races: 31% of the population is younger than 15 years compared with 21% of the US population as a whole. Additionally, 6% of the AIAN population is over 65 years of age compared with the US population as a whole at 12% (IHS 2003).

The underreporting and racial misclassification of AIAN persons in national, state, and local data has been a consistent problem (Epstein et al. 1997, Graber et al. 2005, Stehr-Green et al. 2002, Frost et al. 1992). In *Adjusting for Miscoding of Indian Race on State Death Certificates*, a 1996 US Department of Health and Human Services publication (IHS 1996), the authors reported that IHS areas with the greatest percentage of inconsistent classification of AIAN status were California (30.4%); Oklahoma City, Oklahoma (28.0%); Bemidji, Minnesota (16.1%); and Nashville, Tennessee (12.1%). The major explanations for racial misclassification are the use of Spanish surnames to determine a person's race and the subjective use of personal observation in completing the race item on the death certificates and other health records (Burhansstipanov and Satter 2000, Mihesuah 1998, Burhansstipanov et al. 1999, Frost et al. 1992, Frost and Shy 1980, Hahn et al. 1992, Hahn 1992, Sugarman et al. 1993, Sugarman et al. 1992). IHS now reports data after adjusting for misclassification or misreporting.

Figure 1.1 illustrates the differences in the 1992 to 1994 infant mortality rates for IHS with adjusting for misclassification; the estimated mortality rate increased, with the greatest differences being a 26% increase in the all-areas IHS rate (from 8.7/1000 to 11.9/1000), and a 203% increase (from 3.6/1000 to 11.0/1000) for California.

Figure 1.2 demonstrates an equally surprising difference when examining the 1992 to 1994 homicide rates. When adjusting for misclassification, the estimated rate increased from 13.4/100,000 to 15.1/100,000 for the IHS (all areas), with significant increases in the California Area (6.7/100,000 to

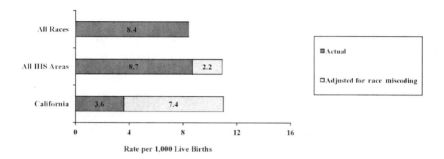

**Figure 1.1. Racial misclassification in 1992-1994 infant mortality rates, United States.**
*Source: IHS 1997.*

11.1/100,000), Oklahoma Area (from 7.1/100,000 to 11.1/100,000), and Bemidji Area (from 11.9/100,000 to 15.5/100,000).

Census data are available on respondents of multiple races for the first time as a direct result of the 1997 Federal Standards on Race and Ethnic Data Collection and Reporting, commonly referred to as Office of Management and Budget 15 (OMB 15). One of the most important issues under OMB 15 is how census and other federal data on persons with multiple races will be tabulated and reported. For the first time, this allows for better data collection on American Indians and other races. OMB 15 now requires data collection for

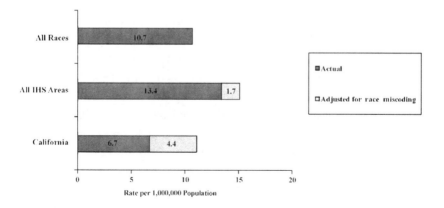

**Figure 1.2. Racial misclassification in homicide death rates, United States.**
*Source: IHS 1997.*

one ethnicity (Latino) and five races (Native Hawaiian and Pacific Islander, American Indian and Alaska Native, Asian or Asian-American, African-American or Black, and White). Additionally, the National Center for Health Statistics and the Census Bureau are the only federal agencies allowed to include "other" as a sixth racial category. At the same time, it is forcing researchers, tribal and urban leaders, and individuals to take a hard look at what it means to be Native in the 21st century.

Data from the National Health Interview Survey for 1993 to 1995 show that 1.6% of respondents reported being more than one race. However, among the respondents who reported AIAN race, greater than 50% also reported at least one other race (Durch and Madans 2001). In the 2000 US Census, approximately 7 million people indicated that they belonged to more than one race, and 40% of these persons reported American Indian or Alaska Native as one of their races. In the 2010 Census, the number of individuals reporting American Indian or Alaska Native alone or in combination with another race was 5.2 million people, with 2.9 million reporting AIAN race alone. This resulted in a 40% increase of multiple-race AIAN persons, compared with 18% increase in the AIAN-only category between 2000 and 2010.

In 2000, 138,696 persons in Los Angeles County reported AIAN race. Of these, 62,000 persons reported at least one additional race. In 2010, however, only 54,236 persons reported AIAN race in combination with an other race and 28,215 persons reported AIAN race alone. In 2010, New York City, New York, reported the largest AIAN population alone or in combination with a population of 111,749 combined. Of those, 57,512 reported AIAN race alone and 54,237 reported AIAN status in combination with another race. The areas with the largest increase in AIAN populations both alone and in combination with other races were in the South with an increase from 31 to 33%. The West declined from 43 to 41%, while still retaining the largest share of AIAN persons, whether alone or in combination with other races. California and Oklahoma still remain as the two states with the largest populations of AIAN alone or in-combination with 14% and 9.2%, respectively. The city with the largest proportion of AIAN persons alone or in combination at 12% was Anchorage, Alaska (US Census 2010).

Another issue of concern is the mislabeling of race/ethnicity in the dissemination of results. For example, researchers frequently use the term American Indian and Alaska Native or Native American in the title and body of their published research. However, the studies may only include persons from one or two tribes. As mentioned previously, data should be reported to the level of specificity allowed through agreement with the tribe or community sampled.

Tabulation and aggregation of data is a growing concern in Indian country. Racial misclassification remains the greatest concern for improving data accuracy, but how researchers tabulate and report multiracial persons is also a problem. The following quote from OMB 15 indicates the opposition to the multiple race category by tribes: "Comments from the American Indian tribal governments also were opposed to the recommendation concerning reporting more than one race" (1997). However, census racial categories and counts are the major organizing tool for public health data (Tashiro 2002). Race and ethnicity are not always mutually exclusive. In the United States the census is presently concerned with only one ethnicity, Latino. Not only is it possible for people to be American Indians and Alaska Natives and Latino, it is quite a common occurrence in the Southwest (Burhansstipanov and Satter 2000). When collapsing race and ethnicity data into one category, AIAN persons should not be aggregated in with Latinos. Ideally, each of the five races should be broken down by Latino and non-Latino classification, providing a more accurate picture of race and ethnic classification.

Unfortunately, states retain the authority to collect and tabulate data in ways that may differ from federal guidelines. California, for example, produces state population estimates and vital statistics by race using a set of mutually exclusive tabulation categories that include Latino/Hispanic along with the race categories specified by OMB. Persons of Latino/Hispanic ethnicity are assigned to the Hispanic category regardless of race.

A common approach in research is to compare data across years and to simplify statistical procedures by recoding persons of more than one race either into a single race category or by leaving them in a "more than one race" category. The latter of the two methods is analogous to an "other" category, which is of no use when attempting to develop and assess public health programs and services. Culturally competent health interventions require specific knowledge of the population of interest that is not captured by an "other" classification.

## AGGREGATING DATA

Most AIAN statistics are reported using the category American Indian and Alaska Native or "other" and are reported at the national, regional, and state levels. There are two reasons for this practice: (1) the sample sizes in national surveys are too small to report tribal specific information, and (2) reporting information for some of the smaller tribes could lead to breaches in confidentiality. However, the 566 federally recognized tribes (US Department of the Interior 2013), the numerous state-recognized tribes, and the numerous self-identified AIAN persons do not belong to one pan-Indian group. While there are similarities among Indigenous groups, there are many cultural, behavioral, and social differences that must be taken into account. Unfortunately, there are not enough specific data to describe the health status of a given tribe or urban Indian community. These data are critical to making informed policy, planning, and resource allocation decisions for improving the health of the population.

There are few methods to reduce racial misreporting, specifically for AIAN persons of more than one race. Various authors recommend using the inclusive count (single and multiple race) of AIAN persons, as it appears to be more appropriate for service planning and outreach; however, even that approach has social, political, and economic implications for AIAN populations (Swan et al. 2006, Burhansstipanov et al. 1999, Stehr-Green et al. 2002, Hahn et al. 1992, Houghton 2002). Federal agencies, including the National Center for Health Statistics, suggest combining single- and multiple-race AIAN persons in the AIAN category (OMB 1997). Still, many statisticians and data users either are unaware of the suggestion or do not understand the implications of other approaches. This has resulted in general ignorance regarding the management of AIAN racial classification in data among researchers. As Houghton stated in his 2002 article on racial misclassification, "the first stage in the process of rectifying the misclassification issue may be the introduction of decolonization and cultural awareness programs for staff."

## SUMMARY

The dramatic historical, political, and social interactions between AIAN communities and the US government have made significant impacts upon the real and perceived health of AIAN populations. Defining and reporting who is

Indian creates further concerns about the data on health status and healthcare and, when used incorrectly, can negatively influence policy and programming. The information in this chapter can help guide researchers in understanding Native concerns about research in general, and data collection, management, and reporting specifically, while drawing attention to the issues of under-reporting and racial misclassification.

## ACKNOWLEDGMENTS

This chapter was written by Delight E. Satter in her private capacity while Director of the American Indian Research Program at the UCLA Center for Health Policy Research. No official support or endorsement by the Centers for Disease Control and Prevention and the Department of Health and Human Services is intended, nor should be inferred.

## REFERENCES

Brookings Institution. 1928. *The Problem of Indian Administration: Report of a Survey Made at the Request of Honorable Hubert Work, Secretary of the Interior, and submitted to him, February 21, 1928.* Baltimore, MD: The Johns Hopkins Press.

Brown ER, Ponce N, Rice T, et al. 2002. *The State of Health Insurance in California: Findings From the 2001 California Health Interview Survey.* Los Angeles: University of California, Los Angeles Center for Health Policy Research.

Bryan RT. 1999. Alien species and emerging infectious diseases: Past lessons and future implications. In: Sandlund OT, Schei PJ, Viken A, editors. *Invasive Species and Biodiversity Management.* Boston, MA: Kluwer Academic Publishers; 163–175.

Burhansstipanov L, Hampton JW, Wiggins C. 1999. Issues in cancer data and surveillance for American Indian and Alaska Native populations. *J Registry Manage.* 26(4): 153–57.

Burhansstipanov L, Satter D. 2000. Office of Management and Budget: racial categories and implications for American Indians and Alaska Natives. *Am J Public Health.* 90(11): 1720–23.

Canby WC. 1998. *American Indian Law in a Nutshell.* St Paul, MN: West Group.

Comptroller of the United States. 1976. *Investigations of Allegations Concerning Indian Health Services*. Washington, DC: Government Printing Office.

DeFine MS. 1997. A history of governmentally coerced sterilization: the plight of the Native American woman. *Native Am Political Issues*. Available at: http://www.oocities.org/capitolhill/9118/mike2.html. Accessed September 15, 2013.

Deloria V, Lytle CM. 1983. *American Indians, American Justice*. Austin: University of Texas Press.

Deloria V, Lytle CM. 1984. *The Nations Within: The Past and Future of American Indian Sovereignty*. Austin: University of Texas Press.

Deloria V, Wilkins DE. 2000. *Tribes, Treaties, and Constitutional Tribulations*. Austin: University of Texas Press.

Dillingham B. 1977. Indian women and IHS sterilization practices. *Am Indian J*. 3(1):27–28.

Dillingham B. 1977. Sterilization of Native Americans. *Am Indian J*. 3(7):16–19.

Dixon M, Roubideaux Y, editors. 2001. *Promises to Keep: Public Health Policy for American Indians and Alaska Natives in the 21st Century*. Washington, DC: American Public Health Association.

Durch JS, Madans JH. 2001. Methodological issues for vital rates and population estimates: 1997 OMB standards for data on race and ethnicity. *Vital Health Stat*. 4(31):1–30.

Epstein M, Moreno R, Bacchetti P. 1997. The underreporting of deaths of American Indian children in California, 1979 through 1993. *Am J Public Health*. 87(8):1363–6.

Frost F, Taylor V, Fries E. 1992. Racial misclassification of Native Americans in a surveillance, epidemiology and end results cancer registry. *Natl Cancer Inst*. 84(12):957–62.

Frost F, Shy KK. 1980. Racial differences between linked birth and infant death records in Washington State. *Am J Public Health*. 70(9):974–76.

General Accounting Office. 1976. Investigation of Allegations Concerning the American Indian Health Service. B-164031 (5); HRD-77-3. Available at: http://www.gao.gov/assets/120/117355.pdf. Accessed July 11, 2013.

Getches DH, Wilkinson CF, Williams RA. 2004. *Cases and Materials on Federal Indian Law.* 5th edition. Eagan, MN: Thomson West.

Graber JM, Corkum BE, Sonnenfeld N, et al. 2005. Underestimation of cardiovascular disease mortality among Maine American Indians: the role of procedural and data errors. *Am J Public Health.* 95(5):827–30.

Grim CW. 2004. Direct services is a self-determination option. Presented at the Direct Service Tribes First Annual Meeting, Phoenix, AZ, June 2, 2004. Available at: http://www.ihs.gov/PublicInfo/PublicAffairs/Director/2004_Statements/Compositor run back onto previous line-Jun_2004.pdf. Accessed October 27, 2010.

Hahn RA, Mulinare J, Teutsch SM. 1992. Inconsistencies in coding of race and ethnicity between birth and death in US infants: a new look at infant mortality, 1983 through 1985. *JAMA.* 267(2):259–63.

Hahn R. 1992. The state of federal health statistics on racial and ethnic groups. *JAMA.* 267(2):268–71.

Holt MI. 2001. *Indian Orphanages.* Lawrence: University Press of Kansas.

Houghton F. 2002. Misclassification of racial/ethnic minority deaths: the final colonization. *Am J Public Health.* 92(9):1386.

*Indian Health Care Improvement Act of 1976.* Public Law 94-437, codified as amended at 25 USC §§ 1601 et seq., and 42 USC §§ 1395qq and 1396j).

Indian Health Service. 1996. *Adjusting for Miscoding of Indian Race on State Death Certificates.* Rockville, MD: Indian Health Service.

Indian Health Service. 1999. *Trends in Indian Health 1998–99.* Rockville, MD: Indian Health Service. Available at: http://www.ihs.gov/publicinfo/publications/trends98/trends98.asp. Accessed December 30, 2012.

Indian Health Service. 2003. *Trends in Indian Health.* Rockville, MD: Indian Health Service.

Indian Health Service. 2011. *Final User Population Memo.* Available at: http://www.ihs.gov/California/uploadedfiles/training/FY2010-MemoFinalUserPop.pdf. Accessed February 19, 2012.

Indian Health Service. Office of Tribal Self Governance. Available at: http://www.ihs.gov/selfgovernance/index.cfm?module=dsp_otsg_about. Accessed September 9, 2013.

Indian Self-Determination and Education Assistance Act of 1975. Public Law 93-638, codified as amended at 25 USC §§ 450a-450n.

Johnson EA, Rhoades ER. 2000. The history and organization of Indian Health Services. In: Rhoades ER, editor. *American Indian Health, Innovations in Healthcare, Promotion and Policy*. Baltimore, MD: The Johns Hopkins Press.

Kickingbird K, Rhoades ER. 2000. The relation of Indian Nations to the US government. In: Rhoades ER, editor. *American Indian Health, Innovations in Healthcare, Promotion and Policy*. Baltimore, MD: The Johns Hopkins Press.

Larson JK. 1977. And then there were none. *Christian Century*. 26:62–63. Available at: http://www.religion-online.org/showarticle.asp?title=1133. Accessed July 12, 2013.

Mihesuah D. 1998. *Natives and Academics: Researching and Writing About American Indians*. Lincoln: University of Nebraska Press.

Mosher WD, Martinez GM, Chandra A, et al. 2004. Use of contraception and use of family planning services in the US, 1982–2002. *Advance Data From Vital and Health Statistics*. No 350. Hyattsville, MD: National Center for Health Statistics.

Nelson SH, Manson SM. 2000. Mental health and mental disorders. In: Rhoades ER, editor. *American Indian Health, Innovations in Healthcare, Promotion and Policy*. Baltimore, MD: The Johns Hopkins Press.

Office of Management and Budget. 1997. *Federal Register Notice October 30, 1997. Revisions to the Standards for the Classification of Federal Data on Race and Ethnicity*. Available at: http://www.whitehouse.gov/omb/fedreg_1997standards. Accessed July 12, 2013.

Perdue T, Green MD, editors. 1995. *The Cherokee Removal: A Brief History With Documents*. Boston, MA: Bedford.

Pevar SL. 1992. *The Rights of Indians and Tribes: The basic ACLU guide to Indian and Tribal Rights*. Carbondale: Southern Illinois University Press.

Pinkerton-Uri C. 1974. Sterilization of young Native women alleged at Indian hospital - 48 operations in July, 1974 alone. *Akwesasne Notes*. 1974:22.

Shelton BL. 2001. Legal and historical basis of Indian healthcare. In: Dixon M, Roubideaux Y, editors. *Promises to Keep: Public Health Policy for American Indian and Alaska Natives in the 21ˢᵗ Century.* Washington, DC: American Public Health Association; 1–28.

*Snyder Act of 1921.* 25 U.S.C 13.

Stehr-Green P, Bettles J, Robertson LD. 2002. Effect of racial/ethnic misclassification of American Indians and Alaskan Natives on Washington State death certificates, 1989–1997. *Am J Public Health.* 92:443–444.

Sugarman JR, Hill G, Forquera R, et al. 1992. Coding of race on death certificates of patients of an urban Indian health clinic, Washington, 1973–1988. *IHS Provid.* July:113–115.

Sugarman JR, Soderberg R, Gordon JE, et al. 1993. Racial misclassification of American Indians: its effect on injury rates in Oregon, 1989 through 1990. *Am J Public Health.* 83(5):681–84.

Swan J, Breen N, Burhansstipanov L, et al. 2006. Cancer screening and risk factor rates among American Indians. *Am J Public Health.* 96(2):340–50.

Tashiro C. 2002. Considering the significance of ancestry through the prism of mixed-race identity. *Adv Nurs Sci.* 25(2):1–21.

Tribalhealthcare.org. 2013. *CMS Announces Tribal Consultation.* Available at: http://tribalhealthcare.org/blog/cms-announces-tribal-consultation. Accessed July 12, 2013.

*Tribal Self-Governance Amendments of 2000.* Public Law 106–260. 25 U.S.C. 458aaa.

US Department of Interior. Bureau of Indian Affairs. Available at: http://www.bia.gov/WhoWeAre/index.htm. Accessed September 11, 2013.

US Census Bureau. 2010. *The American Indian and Alaska Native Population: 2010.* Available at: http://www.census.gov/prod/cen2010/briefs/c2010br-10.pdf. Accessed July 12, 2013.

US Senate Committee on Indian Affairs. 2010. *How The Patient Protection and Affordable Care Act Will Help Native Americans.* Available at: http://www.indian.senate.gov/news/pressreleases/upload/PPACAforIndianHealthCare2.pdf. Accessed July 12, 2013.

Verano JW, Ubelaker DH. 1991. Health and disease in the Pre-Columbian world. In: Sandlund OT, Schei PJ, Viken A, editors. *Invasive Species and Biodiversity Management.* Washington, DC: Smithsonian Institution Press.

Volscho TW. 2009. *Sterilization Racism: A Quantitative Study of Pan-Ethnic and Other Ethnic Disparities in Sterilization, Sterilization Regret, and Long-Acting Contraceptive Use* [dissertation]. Storrs: University of Connecticut.

Wilkins DE, Lomawaima KT. 2001. *Uneven Ground: American Indian Sovereignty and Federal Law.* Norman: University of Oklahoma Press.

Wissow LS. 2000. Suicide among American Indians and Alaska Natives. In: Rhoades ER, editor. *American Indian Health, Innovations in Healthcare, Promotion and Policy.* Baltimore, MD: The Johns Hopkins Press.

Zuckerman S, Haley J, Roubideaux Y, et al. 2004. Health service access, use, and insurance coverage among American Indians/Alaska natives and Whites: what role does the Indian play? *Am J Public Health.* 94(1):53–9.

Self-Governance Education and Communication. Available at: http://www.tribalselfgov. org/red%20book/the%20history%20&%20goals/history_of_the_tribal_self.htm. Accessed September 9, 2013.

# 2

# Overview of Epidemiology and Public Health Data in Native American Populations

Teshia G. Arambula Solomon, PhD, and Leslie L. Randall, RN, MPH, BSN

## INTRODUCTION

### Overcoming Invisibility Through Data

The dramatic historical, political, and social relationships between Native American (NA) communities and tribal nations and the US government discussed in Chapter 1 and similar experiences of Native Hawaiian and Canadian Aboriginals has made a significant impact upon the real and perceived health of Native peoples in the Americas and elsewhere. While traditional Native stories tell of difficulty prior to colonization in living a life that was closely connected to the earth and ecosystem, they also include tales of prosperity and good health (Smylie 2013). Measuring the impact of colonization and policies of assimilation and annihilation is often limited due to the lack of complete health data on some of the affected communities. It is clear, however, that colonization has had a critical influence on the health of Indigenous populations (World Heath Organization [WHO] 2007), and the resultant effect on NA economic and social structures have left them a poor minority living among an economically prosperous majority (Smylie 2013).

### Health Disparities in Native American Populations

While striking health disparities have been found in many areas of healthcare and disease, a sophisticated, systematic population-level tracking system does not exist (Smylie 2010). The lack of community-specific national health surveillance systems for Native Americans in Canada and the United States that exists for the majority inhibits the delivery of evidence-based public health interventions that would reduce morbidity and mortality.

This chapter discusses the complexity of describing the health of NA populations and the published information on the health disparities experienced by NA communities in North America, including Pacific Islanders. While an estimated 5.2 million US citizens self-reported AIAN race alone or in combination with another race in the 2010 Census, with about 3.7 million of them living in urban communities (UIHI 2013), defining who is and is not AIAN is problematic. There are 566 federally recognized and more than 100 state-recognized tribal nations (tribes, nations, bands, pueblos, communities, rancherias, and native villages) in the United States, but those numbers do not account for the descendants of tribes that have been lost or are not officially recognized. It also does not take into account each AIAN tribal or community group's definition of membership.

The Asian/Pacific Islander population (API) and the term Native Hawaiian and other Pacific Islanders (NHOPI) refers to descendants of the original Natives of Hawai'i, Guam, Samoa, or other Pacific Islands. While the aggregation of these racial categories provides a population size of a magnitude necessary for finding statistical significance, it limits the capacity to provide detailed information, specifically for the NHOPI subgroups. This is particularly relevant given the rapid growth of some of these populations: as of the 2010 Census, 1.2 million NHOPI persons of either sole or combined race living in the United States were identified as one of the fastest growing subpopulations (Hixson et al. 2010). Three politically and culturally distinct groups constitute the reported 1,172,785 Aboriginal peoples of Canada: First Nations (FN; 698,025), Inuit (50,480), and Métis (389,780; Statistics Canada 2008b). Aboriginal peoples are the fastest growing and youngest population in Canada, with a 45% increase in population growth over the decade between 1996 and 2006 compared with an 8% increase for the non-Aboriginal population (Statistics Canada 2008b).

The current understanding of health status and healthcare of the NA population is incomplete. Defining, identifying, and reporting who is a Native American creates concerns about the data on health status and healthcare. In addition, patterns of risk behavior, disease status, and healthcare access vary among urban, rural, and remote communities; across geographical regions; between men and women; and across socioeconomic strata. Therefore, it is important to critically examine descriptions of the health status of these populations and to understand the limitations inherent in how data are collected, who is involved, and who or what is excluded. Additionally, data on NA populations are so scarce that many tribal nations, NA communities, and researchers have to rely on data that may be a decade old.

## UNEQUAL PATTERNS IN DEATH AND DISEASE

### *Morbidity and Mortality*

Improvements in the health status of Native Americans have been measured in the areas of infectious diseases, injury, alcoholism, chronic liver disease, and overall mortality and life expectancy (Berry 2004, Ring 2003). However, not all areas, or NA people, benefit equally—for example, while there have been improvements in treatment for infectious diseases in most age groups, this does not hold true for older AIAN adults (Holman 2001). Also, health disparities in care for AIAN people with both chronic and infectious diseases still exist.

Life expectancy rates indicate that an AIAN person will die on average 4.1 years earlier (age 73.6 years) than the average US person (age 77.7 years; IHS 2013). In 2005, chronic liver disease was the sixth leading cause of death for American Indians and Alaska Natives, but was not even ranked in the top 10 for the White, Black, or API populations. See Table 2.1 for comparisons of mortality rates for Native Americans in the United States.

Leading causes of death for NHOPI persons include cancer, heart disease, unintentional injuries (accidents), stroke, and diabetes (CDC/OMH 2013). Additionally, the tuberculosis rate (cases per 100,000) in 2010 was eight times higher for NHOPI persons, with a case rate of 16.6 as compared with 2.0 for the White population. According to Panapasa et al. (2010), Native Hawaiians experience higher mortality rates than do non-Hispanic Whites in older age groups, but the same gap also appears at mid-life. In the United States, NHOPI

Table 2.1. Comparisons of Mortality Rates for Native American Groups in the United States

| | AIAN 2004–2006 | NHOPI 2007 | US All Races 2005 | AIAN:US All Races Ratio |
|---|---|---|---|---|
| All causes | 980.0 | | 798.8 | 1.2 |
| Alcohol-induced | 43.0 | | 7.0 | 6.1 |
| Breast cancer | 21.0 | 33.53 | 24.1 | 0.9 |
| Cerebrovascular/stroke | 46.6 | 57.1 | 46.6 | 1.0 |
| Cervical cancer | 3.3 | 18.1[a] | 2.4 | 1.4 |
| Diabetes | 68.1 | | 24.6 | 2.8 |
| Heart disease | 206.2 | 44.34 | 211.1 | 1.0 |
| HIV infection | 3.0 | | 4.2 | 0.7 |
| Homicide (assault) | 11.7 | | 6.1 | 1.9 |
| Infant deaths[b] | 8.0 | | 6.9 | 1.2 |
| Malignant neoplasms | 176.2 | | 183.8 | 1.0 |
| Maternal deaths | 16.9 | | 15.1 | 1.1 |
| Pneumonia/influenza | 27.1 | | 20.3 | 1.3 |
| Suicide | 19.8 | | 10.9 | 1.8 |
| Tuberculosis | 1.2 | | 0.2 | 6.0 |
| Unintentional injuries[c] | 93.8 | | 39.1 | 2.4 |

Notes: AIAN=American Indians and Alaska Natives; NHOPI=Native Hawaiians and Other Pacific Islanders.
Sources: Hawai State Dept. of Health 2007, Miller et al. 2008, Henderson et al. 2007, IHS 2013.
[a]For the Samoan population.
[b]Infant deaths per 1,000 live births.
[c]Includes motor vehicle crashes.

persons also suffer from a number of health disparities when compared with non-Hispanic Whites, including a 2.5 times higher diabetes rate, a roughly 60% higher infant mortality rate (9.1 vs 5.7/1,000), and a twofold-higher hepatitis B (3.0 vs 1.3/100,000) and asthma rate. Data on risk behaviors also indicate that compared with other populations, NHOPI persons experience higher rates of smoking, alcohol consumption, and obesity (CDC 2009).

The leading causes of death among FN persons are similar to that of other Canadian citizens, but health disparities include a suicide rate among the Inuit that is six times higher than that for the rest of the Canadian population (Reading 2009). Improvements in life expectancy also lag for Native populations in Canada. The age-standardized death rate among the registered FN population in Western Canada (5.3/100,000 population/year) is more than double the age-standardized death rate among the corresponding general

Canadian population (2.4 per 100,000 population/year). For the registered FN population, the 2001 life expectancy rate remaining at age 25 years was lower than that of the general Canadian population by 5.7 years for males and 6.8 years for females despite a narrowing of the gap between populations by 40% from 1991 to 2006 (Health Canada 2002, Tjepkema et al. 2009). The other part of the health picture of the FN population show that they experience disproportionately high rates of tuberculosis, diabetes, injuries, suicide, and cardiovascular disease (Reading 2009, Assembly of First Nations/FNIGC 2007, Health Canada 2005, Health Canada 2009). Métis adults also have a lower life expectancy compared with non-Aboriginal adults, and age-standardized mortality rates for Métis are reported as significantly higher compared with that of the non-Aboriginal population (Tjepkema et al. 2009). Métis adults were more likely to report being diagnosed with arthritis or rheumatism, high blood pressure, asthma, and diabetes compared with the general Canadian population (Janz et al. 2009).

*Infant Mortality*

Infant health and deaths are an important indicator of the health of a population. Infant mortality is the risk of death during the first year of life and is influenced by the mother's health, behavioral practices, and external factors, including socioeconomic conditions and access to pre- and postnatal healthcare. Leading causes of death during the neonatal period (<28 days of life) include premature birth, low birthweight, and congenital malformations. The leading causes of infant deaths during the first 28 days through 11 months of life (postneonatal) are Sudden Infant Death Syndrome (SIDS) and congenital malformations (Heron and Smith 2003).

Significant disparities between Native and non-Native infant mortality have been found in Canada and the United States (Smylie et al. 2010). Data presented by the CDC show that infant mortality rates for AIAN persons for 2009 (8.47/1,000 live births) were higher than the US average (6.39/1,000; Mathews and MacDorman 2012). In 2002, the infant mortality rate for Native Hawaiians was 9.6 per 1,000 live births, higher than the rate for all populations combined (7.0/1,000). Neonatal mortality rates for these populations for the same time period show a disparity between Native Hawaiians (5.6/1,000 live births) and the US average (4.6), but not for AIAN persons (4.6), while the postneonatal rates show rates almost twice as high for both AIAN and Native

Hawaiian populations at 4.0 per 1,000 live births compared with the US average of 2.3 (Health US 2007).

Mortality rates vary from state to state. For example, rates for infants of AIAN mothers ranged from a high of 23.9 per 1,000 live births in Mississippi and a low of 7.29 per 1,000 live births in New Mexico for 2005 to 2007 (Matthews and McDorman 2011). Additionally, leading causes of infant death in the United States vary by race/ethnicity of the mother; congenital malformation rates were 1.48 times higher, SIDS rates were 2.4 times higher, and the unintentional injury rate was 2.3 times higher for infants born to AIAN women than for those born to non-Hispanic White women (Matthews and McDorman 2011).

In the Aberdeen Area of the IHS, which includes North and South Dakota, Nebraska, and Iowa, the infant mortality rate was 12.5 per 1,000 live births in 2010. This is 74% higher than the general US population rate and 40% higher than the general IHS rate. The neonatal mortality rate in the Aberdeen Area for 1996 to 1998 was 5.6 times higher, while the postneonatal mortality was 6.9 times higher than that of the general US population (DHHS 2005). The SIDS rate in Aberdeen was 27.6 per 1,000 live births, marking a 158% increase over the general US population rate and a 52% increase over the general IHS rate (Eaglestaff et al. 2005). An eight-year review of Aberdeen Area infant mortality found that a large percentage of the deaths were attributable to SIDS (28%), premature births (24%), and lack of prenatal care (38%); nearly two-thirds of the deaths (62%) were male infants (Eaglestaff et al. 2006). In response to their findings, the study authors recommended grief counseling for parents, families, and day care providers, enhanced and very early prenatal care, especially for women who had previously experienced an infant death, and genetic consultation for families of children found to have congenital malformations (Eaglestaff et al. 2007).

In Canada, data on FN infant deaths are incomplete and do not, therefore, provide a nation-wide picture of this group's infant mortality rates. Available regional data, however, show infant mortality rates to be about twice that of non-Aboriginal rates (Smylie et al. 2010). Infant mortality rates for FN persons were 2.3 times higher in rural areas and 2.1 times higher in urban areas than those of the non-FN population in British Columbia, while all-location postneonatal mortality rates were 3.6 times as high (Luo et al. 2004a). Disparities were also found in the province of Manitoba, with FN infant mortality rates twice as high for FN persons; postneonatal mortality rates for

FN persons were 3.6 times higher (Luo et al. 2010). Infant mortality rates among the Inuit have consistently been found to be four times the total Canadian rate (Luo et al. 2004b). In terms of cause, there are a disproportionate number of deaths of Aboriginal infants due to congenital abnormalities (Luo et al. 2010, Statistics Canada 2008a), respiratory tract infections, and SIDS (Luo et al. 2004a, Luo et al. 2010, Luo et al. 2004b).

*Morbidity*

The connection between morbidity and mortality is not as obvious as it would seem. Many Native people suffer not only from one disease state but often from multiple co-morbidities, compounded by the social determinants of health including poverty, poor access to healthcare, and the stress of life, both past and present. For example, while injury may be the cause of death on a death certificate, many factors may have contributed to the cause. Was an automobile accident a result of alcohol- or drug-impaired driving or was it because of unlit, poorly marked, and dangerous reservation road conditions, or both? Was a cervical cancer death caused by infections acquired over a lifetime of sexual abuse, or an undiagnosed or untreated condition? Documenting the health status of Native populations and analyzing and addressing the contributing factors within a socioecological framework is critical. Of the most pressing health conditions facing Native populations, which of these are the results of poverty, a lifetime of abuse, neglect, racism, isolation, or ineffectual policies and programs and extreme underfunding of both healthcare and education? Native Americans, particularly children, and in fact Indigenous people worldwide, suffer disproportionately from certain health conditions, and the need to understand and have an impact on such conditions is crucial for the well-being of Native nations. There are some disparities so great that they demand not only attention but also action.

## HEALTH CONDITIONS REQUIRING URGENT ATTENTION

### Diabetes

Diabetes mellitus is a persistent and growing problem among Native Americans. When compared with the US non-Hispanic White population, the prevalence of diabetes is 16.5% higher among AIAN persons. Native Hawaiians and other Pacific Islanders specifically have been found to have the highest percentage of diabetes (20.6% age adjusted), three times that of the non-Hispanic White population (6.8%) and double that of Latino persons (11.1%; Asian and Pacific Islander Health Forum 2010). The US National Health and Nutrition Examination Survey (NHANES) II found that age-adjusted type 2 diabetes prevalence was four times as high in two rural Hawaiian communities as in the average participant (Grandinetti et al. 1998). This is not a new phenomenon—in fact, the high prevalence of diabetes among Native Hawaiians has been documented since the 1960s (Grandinetti et al. 1998, Sloan 1963). The prevalence of type 2 diabetes mellitus among NA youth has more than doubled between 1994 and 2004 and has quadrupled in some NHOPI subgroups (API Health Forum 2010). Particularly high diabetes prevalence has also been found in Micronesian communities (16.2%) and among NHOPIs who have adopted a more westernized lifestyle (Chiem et al. 2006, Collins et al. 1994, Okihiro and Harrigan 2005).

Diabetes is also a health concern in Canada, though prevalence is influenced by heritage, tribe/language group, culture, and geographic location (Delisle et al. 1985). Reported rates are variable; the 2002-2003 Regional Health Survey reported that 19.7% of FN persons had been diagnosed with diabetes and Bobet (1998) found that 6.4% of reserve-living and 8.5% of off-reserve FN persons reported diabetes.

## Mental Health

Information on mental health is lacking for all populations except when a specific type of problem draws special attention. For example, AIAN adults have been found to report more serious psychological distress than other racial and ethnic groups for panic disorder, post-traumatic stress disorder (PTSD), and anxiety disorders (Barnes 2005, Beals 2005). Mental health data are also often presented in discussion of other issues such as substance abuse or homelessness. Almost 20% of NHOPI adults have reported being diagnosed with a depressive disorder compared with 17.4% for AIAN and 15.9% for non-Hispanic White adults; nearly 16% reported an anxiety disorder compared with 17.5% of AIAN and 12.8% of non-Hispanic White persons (APIHF 2010). In the general population, women generally report more depression and anxiety than men, but the opposite was found among the NHOPI population (32% of men vs 5.58% of women for a diagnosed depressive disorder and

19.9% of men vs 10.7% of women for a diagnosed anxiety disorder; APIHF 2010).

The 2000–2001 Canadian Community Health Survey showed that 13.2% of Aboriginals living off-reserve reported a major depressive episode in the past year (1.8 times that of the non-Aboriginal rate) and similar rates were found despite differences in household incomes (Tjepkema 2002). The Regional Health Survey (RHS), however, found dramatically higher depression rates among FN people, with 30.1% of adults and 27.2% of youth reporting feeling sad, blue, or depressed for a period of two weeks or more in the year prior to the survey (First Nations Centre 2005).

Reading (2009) notes that mental health issues among the homeless are rarely discussed but important because of the strong correlation between homelessness and mental illness. Street Health (2007) found that among Aboriginal homeless persons, 16% reported depression, 11% anxiety, 11% addiction to drugs or alcohol, 7% bipolar or manic-depressive disorder, 6% PTSD, and 6% panic disorder.

It is common for patients who suffer from chronic conditions to also suffer from depression. For example, because the rates of diabetes are so high in the NA population, it is not surprising that related depression would also be disproportional.

## Suicide

The facts around suicide attempts and completion are sorrowful for any population, but the reported suicide rates among Indigenous peoples of North America are unfathomable. In the United States in 2007, suicide was the 11th leading cause of death for all ages and the second leading cause of death for AIAN persons between the ages of 15 to 34 years (CDC 2009). Data from the 2009 Youth Risk Behavior Surveillance Survey show 13.8% of US youth reported considering suicide and 6.3% reported attempting suicide at least once in the previous 12 months (CDC 2009). Death by suicide for AIAN children aged 10 to 14 years is more than triple the national rates (27.72 compared with 8.5/100,000 persons; CDC 2009). Among persons aged 15 to 24 years, there are an estimated 100 to 200 attempts for every completed suicide (Goldsmith et al. 2002). In Canada, suicide among registered FN persons in Western Canada accounts for greater premature mortality than either circulatory diseases or cancers (Health Canada 2002).

Of all the suicides in the United States that were tested for substances consumed at the time of death, one-third tested positive for alcohol or other illegal substances at the time of death (Karch 2012). Data from 2005 and 2006 show that alcohol use was evident with most completed suicides among AIAN persons over 10 years of age. For all decedents tested, AIAN persons aged 30 to 39 years had the highest percentage of persons with blood alcohol over the legal limit at 54.3%, while those aged 20 to 29 years showed alcohol levels at 50.0%; levels for all other races were much lower. It is important to keep in mind that these may not truly be representative, given the aforementioned issues of underestimating the problem due to issues of racial misclassification (CDC MMWR 2009).

The suicide attempt rate among NHOPIs was twice as high as that among non-Hispanic Whites from 1999 to 2005 (CDC 2009). Eleven to 13% of Native Hawaiian high school students reported attempting suicide one or more times in the previous year (2009 YRBS, Yuen et al. 2000).

In Micronesia, Guam, and Western Samoa, researchers have found that suicide completion rates increase sharply from adolescence to young adulthood, and then drop with the 30-year age group on (Booth 1999; Else et al. 2007). In the United States, NHOPI and AIAN adolescents had the highest percentages of having seriously considered attempting suicide (19.2% and 19.0%, respectively) and of having made a plan about how they would attempt suicide (13.2% and 17.0%, respectively; YRBS 2009).

Among FN youth, 9.6% reported attempts of suicide and 21% reported suicide ideation (Assembly Of First Nations 2007). Of FN adults, 31% report having had suicidal thoughts, while 15% report attempts (18.5% of men vs 13% of women; RHS Quick Facts 2007).

## Substance Abuse

The Substance Abuse and Mental Health Services Administration (SAMHSA) reported that 8.7% of the US population aged 12 years and over are current users of drugs (including alcohol), compared with 18.3% of the AIAN population, with the unemployed reporting the highest rates of use (SAMHSA 2010). Patterns of alcohol use among AIAN youth appear to be similar to those of non-Hispanic White youth (YRBS 2009). National data indicate that alcohol use among NHOPI high school students is comparatively low; 68% have tried alcohol, 34.8% currently drink, and 20.6% drink heavily (White students report

74%, 44.7%, and 27.8%, respectively, and AIAN students report 74%, 42.8%, and 29.9% respectively; CDC 2009). However, marijuana use was higher among NHOPI (40.5% lifetime, 24.8% current) and AIAN (50.8%, 31.6%) adolescents when compared with their White counterparts (36.8%, 31.6%; CDC 2009). Reported illicit drug use (including cocaine, heroin, methamphetamines) among NA high school students is also very high (CDC 2009). Among adolescents in the United States, 18.3% of AIAN and 10.1% of NHOPI individuals reported using one or more forms of cocaine ever compared with 6.7% of the White youth (CDC 2011). Heroin use is about three times as high for NHOPI youth (11.1%) as it is for Blacks (2.7%), almost four times as high as for Hispanics (3.3%), and three times that of AIAN youth (4.3%) (CDC 2011). Methamphetamine use by NHOPI teens (6.7%) and AIANs (7.1%) is almost double that of non-Hispanic White teens (3.7%; CDC 2011).

First Nations people of Canada report that they are more likely to abstain completely from alcohol (34.4%) and report a lower frequency of alcohol consumption (17.8% consume less than 1 drink per week) than non-FN respondents (20.7% and 44%, respectively). Unfortunately, FN people also report that they are more likely to be heavy drinkers (defined as having more than five drinks on a single occasion) and doing so on a weekly basis more frequently (16% FN persons vs 6.2% non-FN persons). Alcohol was related to 6.4% of injuries and 27.1% of assaults against FN youth and 23.5% of "status" Indian[1] deaths with other drugs attributing to 6.2% of status Indian deaths (First Nations Centre 2005).

Over one-quarter of FN individuals reported marijuana use, with males aged 18 to 29 years (29.1%) reporting daily use of marijuana. Illicit drug use has been found to be twice that among the FN population (7.3%) when compared with the general Canadian population (3%), and is correlated with lower education levels. Substance abuse reported in the 2002–2003 RHS (First

---

[1]An individual recognized by the federal government as being "registered" under the *Indian Act* is referred to as a Registered Indian, or "status" Indian. Status Indians are entitled to a wide range of programs and services offered by federal and provincial governments. Over the years, there have been many rules for deciding who is eligible for registration. Important changes were made to the act in June 1985, when Parliament passed Bill C-31, *An Act to Amend the Indian Act*, to bring it in line with the *Canadian Charter of Rights and Freedoms*, and again in 2011 with the coming into force of Bill C-3, *Gender Equity in Indian Registration Act*. See http://laws.justice.gc.ca/eng/acts/I-5/ and http://www.aadnc-aandc.gc.ca/eng/1100100032374/1100100032378 for more information.

Table 2.2. Native American Substance Abuse Patterns

| | Percent Reporting Use | | | | |
| --- | --- | --- | --- | --- | --- |
| | US White | AIAN | NHOPI | CFN | Canada General Population |
| Ever tried alcohol | 74.0 | 74.0 | 68.0 | - | 89.7 |
| Current drinker | 44.7 | 42.8 | 34.8 | 40.0 | 78.0 |
| Drink heavily | 27.8 | 29.9 | 20.6 | 16.0 | 6.2 |
| Ever used marijuana | 36.8 | 50.8 | 40.5 | 32.7 | 39.4 |
| Current marijuana use | 31.6 | 31.6 | 24.8 | 29.1 | 9.1 |
| Cocaine use | 6.0 | 11.0 | 8.5 | 7.3 | 3.0 |
| Methamphetamine use | 3.5 | 11.0 | 7.7 | | |
| Heroin use | - | 3.1 | 6.0 | | |

Notes: AIAN=American Indian and Alaska Native; CFN=Canada First Nations; NHOPI=Native Hawaiians and Other Pacific Islanders. Dash indicates that no data are available.
Sources: CDC YRBS 2009, First Nations Longitudinal Survey 2002–03, CADUMS 2011.

Nations Centre 2005) found that while the majority of FN youth are nonusers of illicit drugs, about 4% of FN youth reported using PCP, acid/LSD/ amphetamines, ecstasy, inhalants, sedatives or downers, cocaine/crack/free-base, or codeine/morphine/opiates. In addition, 32.7% reported marijuana use. Illicit drug use was related to dependence on alcohol or other substances such as cocaine or marijuana as a "base drug." The survey also found that nonusers reported a higher level of social support. See Table 2.2 for substance abuse patterns for Native Americans.

## Sexual Health

According to the 2010 Youth Risk Behavior Survey, 53.6% of NHOPI and 69% of AIAN high school students reported having had sexual intercourse compared with 44.3% of non-Hispanic White high school students. Additionally, 18.4% of NHOPI and 21.9% of AIAN respondents reported having more than four sexual partners in their lifetime compared with 13.1% of non-Hispanic White students (CDC 2011).

While pregnancy rates for women between the ages of 14 to 19 years are declining overall in the United States, the rates for AIAN peoples (55.5/1,000) are double that of non-Hispanic White women (25.6/1,000; Martin et al. 2010).

Despite these higher rates, more detailed regional, state, and tribe-specific information is limited. In a review of teen childbearing patterns among American Indians and Alaska Natives, Wingo et al. (2011) found that birth rates per 1,000 women aged 14 to 19 years varied geographically, from 24.35 (California) to 123.24 (Aberdeen). In 2007 in the United States, there were 8956 births to AIAN girls aged 15 to 19 years and 121 to AIAN girls younger than 15 years (Wingo et al. 2011). Rutman et al. (2008) reported AIAN urban youth experienced first intercourse prior to age 13 years at a rate triple that of their non-Native counterparts, and Kaufman et al. (2007) found that 32% of AIAN women aged 16 to 18 years had been pregnant at least once.

Factors that put teenage girls at risk for pregnancy also put them at risk for other health issues including sexually transmitted infections (STIs), subsequent pregnancies, initiation of sex at an early age, drinking at an early age, and problems with school (Mead and Ickovics 2005). Data indicate that AIAN adolescents have higher rates of sexual risk behaviors than do other racial/ethnic minority youth (CDC 2009, Hellerstadt et al. 2006, Kaufman 2007, Rutman et al. 2008). AIAN young adults have been found to be less likely to use condoms or other methods of contraception (National Campaign to Prevent Teen and Unplanned Pregnancy 2008) and areas found to have high teen birth rates also have high rates of STIs for teens (CDC 2009). In some areas, chlamydia and gonorrhea rates for AIAN individuals aged 15 to 19 years were three times that of non-Hispanic Whites; syphilis rates were 1.5 times higher (CDC 2009).

The CDC reports STI rates for Native Hawaiians and other Pacific Islanders aggregated with the Asian population. The 2010 reported cases among API for chlamydia, gonorrhea, and syphilis are low in comparison with those for other groups (CDC 2012).

First Nations youth have been found to be more sexually active than are their non-Aboriginal counterparts. As of 2002–2003, nearly 33% of FN youth were sexually active; 20% of those individuals reported use of the birth control pill and 81% reported using a condom, but 10% reported not using any form of contraception. Fewer than 5% of RHS 2002–2003 youth respondents reported ever having been pregnant or being responsible for getting someone pregnant (First Nations Centre 2005).

One study found alarming results that the rate of commercial sex industry exploitation of Aboriginal children and youth is more than 90% in some communities, despite the fact that Aboriginals represent less than 10% of the population. This serious over-representation of Aboriginal youth in the sex trade is believed to be directly linked to extreme poverty and other socioecological factors faced by Aboriginal children and their families (Ontario Federation of Indian Friendship Centres 2004).

## Hidden Areas of Need

### Urban Natives

Few aggregate data sets exist for Native Americans that provide a clear picture of the health status of this varied population living throughout North America. When it comes to health data, racial misclassification has been a well-documented problem, specifically for those living in urban areas. Some data sources and studies fail to ask for racial classification and others fail to report findings for AIAN persons due to the small sample size. Few national data sets have sample sizes large enough to help draw meaningful conclusions and when they do, results from these studies are reflective only of the respondents and may not reflect urban AIAN issues. Conversely, studies conducted with an urban Indian population may not be representative of a specific tribal community's issues. For example, smoking rates vary across regions in the United States—while high in the Plains region, rates are low in the Southwest (Bliss et al. 2008). This may be a reflection of smoking patterns of urban AIAN communities compared with reservation communities and may be influenced by issues of access or income or social acceptance of cigarette smoking. Differential causation remains unclear.

Certain segments of the AIAN population living in urban areas are often transient, returning frequently to tribal homelands for a variety of reasons that include accessing healthcare or other resources. Others may have less contact with their tribal homelands but continue to practice their traditional ways or engage in cultural activities with other urbanized AIAN persons. Still others are quite removed from their ancestral practices and identify socially and culturally with their urban neighbors. Self-identification is at the heart of how AIAN persons view their place in society; some of this identification is defined by blood quantum level or enrollment in a specific tribe. As mentioned in Chapter 1, criteria for tribal membership varies enormously by tribe, and can involve place of residence, language spoken, blood quantum level, proof of descendency, or some combination thereof. As a result of this complexity, describing health information can be challenging. Including urban Indians

Table 2.3. Health Disparities in Urban American Indian and Alaska Natives in the United States

| Health Indicator | Healthy People 2010 | AIAN | Disparity Ratio |
|---|---|---|---|
| SIDS death rate[a] | 0.25 | 1.5 | 6.0 |
| Live births who did not receive early and adequate prenatal care,[b] % | 10.0 | 39.4 | 3.9 |
| Infant death rate[a] | 1.2 | 4.3 | 3.6 |
| Prenatal care later than first trimester, % | 10.0 | 30.7 | 3.1 |
| Uninsured adults aged 18–64 years, % | 1.0[c] | 28.8 | 28.8 |

*Notes:* AIAN=American Indian and Alaska Native; SIDS=Sudden Infant Death Syndrome.
*Source:* Urban Indian Health Institute 2009.
[a]Per 1,000 live births.
[b]Kotelchuck index.
[c]Rounded to 1 from 0 in order to calculate ratio.

with rural reservation populations may skew the data and distort information such as income and access to care, since there are more healthcare options in cities than there are in rural and remote areas. At the same time, having a healthcare center nearby does not ensure accessibility, as finances may prevent individuals from utilizing such resources.[2]

Several selected studies of health disparities in urban communities between AIAN and White persons in the United States show higher rates of low birthweight, risk factors for poor birth outcomes, communicable diseases, mortality among nonelderly individuals, injuries, and alcohol-related deaths among urban Natives (Table 2.3). Other key health problems also exist. For example, SIDS is the leading cause of infant mortality in urban US Natives and is over six times the rate for the general population. Mortality rates for the leading causes of death are lower in urban Natives than in the overall AIAN population, with the exception of alcohol and drug related deaths. However, rates of diabetes, chronic liver disease, cirrhosis, unintentional injuries, and infant mortality are still higher than in the general population (Castor 2006).

Data on urban Aboriginals in Canada, often referred to as "off-reserve" Aboriginals, are very limited; however, the urban community has been found to be significantly disadvantaged compared with their non-Aboriginal counterparts and are twice as likely to live in poverty (Reading 2010). Also,

[2]See http://www.ihs.gov/ihm/index.cfm?module=dsp_ihm_pc_p2c6#2-6.3 for information on patient registration for the IHS.

while urban Aboriginals in Canada constitute only 1.5% of the urban population, they account for 3.4% of the poor population (Lee 2000). Specific health concerns for urban Aboriginals include household mold and air quality (Beavis et al. 1997); diabetes rates have been found to be higher among urban and acculturated Aboriginal peoples (Daniel et al. 1995), as have rates of cardiovascular disease (Yusuf et al. 2001) and arthritis, which has been found to be particularly high among adult women aged 65 years and older (70% of Aboriginal women vs 50% of their Canadian counterparts; Health Canada 2003). These health issues should be considered as well as the issues in homelessness and mental health previously discussed.

## HIV/AIDS

The CDC (2013) reports a rate per 100,000 for diagnosis of HIV infection for NHOPI persons (15.3) that is more than double that for White Americans (7.0), while the rate for AIAN individuals (9.3) is 30% higher than for their non-Hispanic White counterparts. At the end of 2009 in the United States and its territories, about 620 NHOPI individuals were estimated to be living with HIV, with an additional 481 persons living with AIDS (CDC 2010). The CDC (2012) reports that between the start of the AIDS epidemic and 2009, an estimated 363 NHOPI persons have died from the disease.

Canadian Aboriginals continue to experience disparities in HIV/AIDS when compared with other Canadians. Between 4300 and 6100 Aboriginal persons were living with HIV/AIDS in Canada in 2008 (8.0% of all prevalent HIV infections), a 24% increase from 2005. In addition, 12.5% of all new infections were attributed to Aboriginal persons, a disproportionately higher percentage given the number of Aboriginal persons in the total Canadian population (3.8%); this rate of new infections was more than three times the non-Aboriginal rate of 3.6 (PHAC 2009). Of the Aboriginal AIDS cases reported through 2006, 73.1% were among First Nations, 7.3% among Métis, and 3.6% among Inuits (PHAC 2007). Men make up the majority of Aboriginal HIV/AIDS cases but Aboriginal women are overrepresented in HIV/AIDS cases compared with non-Aboriginal women (PHAC 2007). Nearly one-third of Aboriginals living with HIV were younger than 30 years (32.4%) compared with 21% of their Canadian counterparts (PHAC 2007). Aboriginal youth are reported to be infected with HIV at a younger age compared with other Canadians (Health Canada 2012).

## Homelessness

Homelessness is characterized as *absolute* (no shelter and may/may not live on the streets), *relative* (those who have physical shelter that does not meet basic health and safety measures), or *at-risk* (those who live day-by-day in their own physical shelter but could be homeless at any time). Homeless persons may rely on emergency shelters, traditional housing, friends, or family (Reading 2009, Hwang 2001). "Couch surfers" is a term attributed to those who move from location to location (Helin 2002). The NA population disproportionately suffers from homelessness, particularly veterans and urban residents (Carson et al. 2007, Hwang 2001, Helin 2002). Factors that put a person or family at risk for homelessness are correlated with a variety of socioeconomic or health issues, including the following (Dappleton Research Team 2003):

- Having rent or a mortgage that exceeds 25% of personal income;
- Suffering from an acute life crisis;
- Earning a household income below the national average;
- Having a lower education level;
- Being denied access to government housing;
- Qualifying for food banks;
- Being engaged in the sex trade;
- Having severe, chronic medical conditions and no ability to pay for care (Hwang 2001); and
- Having mental health problems or a chronic mental illness (Folsom et al. 2005).

Being homeless puts people at risk for exposure to the elements, poor nutrition, a lack of social support, poor access to healthcare, and stigmatization (Dappleton Research Team 2003).

**American Indians and Alaska Natives.** In the United States, AIAN persons are overrepresented among the homeless, making up 4% of the homeless population but only 1% of the population (US Conference of Mayors 2006). AIAN veterans comprise a significant portion of this group, such that they are overrepresented by approximately 19% (Kasprow and Rosenheck 1998).

A report on homeless NA persons in the United States notes that they often experience discrimination in securing affordable housing whether they choose to live on or off reservation. For US Native Americans, time spent on low-income rental unit waiting lists averages 41 months—twice the national average—despite an estimated 40% of the units being inadequate. For example, 20% of households in tribal areas lack complete plumbing and a third are overcrowded, at a rate over six times the national average (Zerger 2004).

Additionally, AIAN homeless persons delay seeking health services for a number of reasons, including a lack of trust in organizations (particularly government-run organizations) an overall shortage of providers in IHS-run facilities, and an even greater shortage of AIAN providers (Zerger 2004).

*Native Hawaiians and Other Pacific Islanders.* A 2006 *New York Times* article describes the crisis of homelessness in Honolulu at that time, estimating that hundreds of homeless occupy the beach areas in Waikiki, the tourist center, but that along the Waianae Coast on the west shore it was estimated that 1,000 to 4,000 homeless persons live in tent communities, a significant portion of whom were Native Americans (Magin 2006, OHA 2006). The Office of Hawaiian Affairs has worked to put solutions in place to alleviate the homelessness crisis at the time including developing emergency shelters. Between 2003 and 2006, the Waianae Coast Comprehensive Center saw a 234% rise in the homeless population it treated (Perez 2006).

Hawai'i has the third highest homelessness rate in the United States, with about 15,000 people per year and 6,000 on any given day, of whom 26% are considered chronically homeless, an increase of 11% between 2010 and 2011 (HICH 2008, H.O.M.E. 2009). Over 4,000 homeless persons live on the island of Oahu, approximately 70% of whom live in shelters (H.O.M.E. 2009). Of these homeless individuals, 42% are estimated to be children and 28% of the homeless are Native Americans. Other Pacific Islanders also are a part of Hawai'i's homeless population using shelter services: Marshallese 7%, Micronesioan 10%, and Other Pacific Islanders 6%; Native Americans constitute another 2% (HSU Report 2012). A growing segment of the Hawaiian homeless population is youth aging out of the foster care system. Additionally, 96,648 individuals (18,623 households) are considered "hidden homeless," a term that describes a situation in which more than one family shares housing accommodations, while another 262,021 individuals (85,267 households) are at risk of homelessness (HICH 2008).

Approximately 14% of homeless Hawaiian adults have jobs that do not pay enough wages to provide for basic necessities (ICH 2008). Hawai'i's housing costs are the fourth highest in the nation, with a median rent that is 50% higher than the national rate, and where more than 75% of low-income households spend more than half of their income on rent (ICH 2008). The collision caused by exceptionally high housing costs, limited space on an island nation, economic recession, and generational poverty creates a crisis in homelessness among the Native peoples of the islands.

A study using data from the H.O.M.E. project (Yamane et al. 2010), a medical education project in Hawai'i, measured the differences in disease patterns between Native and non-Native Hawaiian homeless on Oahu. They found higher rates of asthma, hypertension, and marijuana and methamphetamine use; lower rates of alcohol use; and no significant difference in illicit drug use. While Native Hawaiians had more visits for diabetes care in the program, the prevalence rates were comparable for non-Native Hawaiians. It is estimated that 20% of Hawai'i's homeless suffer some mental illness (HICH 2008).

***Canadian Aboriginals.*** While the Aboriginal population makes up 2% of the Toronto population, they comprise 25% of the homeless there (Wente 2000). Street Health (2007) listed six common mental health diagnoses reported by Aboriginal homeless persons including: (1) depression (16%), (2) anxiety and addiction to drugs/alcohol (11%), (3) bipolar disorder (7%), and (4) PTSD and panic disorder (6%).

While communities and state and federal government agencies have enacted programs to prevent and end homelessness, multiple support services are needed to help NA veterans, youth, adults, and families stay in housing, including education services and culturally competent and effective approaches to working with NA populations.

## PROBLEMS AND SOLUTIONS IN DATA COLLECTION, STEWARDSHIP, AND SYSTEMS

Smylie et al. (2011) submit that population-based data and data systems should be recast as social resources that contribute to the social, economic, and health of Indigenous populations.

### Improve Data Collection

Weissman and Hasnain (2011) discuss the importance of improving data collection to advance healthcare equity. They posit that improving healthcare data identification of race and ethnicity improves monitoring, identification, and targeting of underlying causes of disparities. Recommendations from the Institute of Medicine (IOM) subcommittee on improving data on race, ethnicity, and language state that, with the improvement of data on patient-provider interactions, healthcare can be improved (2009). More specifically, the report states that by thoroughly understanding causal relationships of specific disparities in health and disease, disparities between groups could be reduced or eliminated.

A report from the Office of the US Assistant Secretary for Planning and Evaluation discusses different data sets and why data collected on American Indians, Alaska Natives, and Native Hawaiians is flawed (McBean 2006, Moy et al. 2006, Westat 2007). Westat (2007) examined the quality of 67 data sets on these groups and found that for all reports, AIANs are often grouped together while Native Hawaiians are often put with other Pacific Islander groups because it provides a larger data set. They also found information on child and elder well-being from the Departments of Justice and Defense and information on policy and transportation were all either missing or limited in scope. Problems resulted from a lack of identification and reporting of race among subgroups and a lack of standardized data collection forms. For example, use of Medicare data is limited when it comes to determining race and ethnicity because information is based on an individual's social security information. Unfortunately, many people received their social security number (SSN) prior to 1980 when only three racial categories were available: Black, White, and Other. Therefore many NAs are perpetually misidentified as "Other" in data sets using SSNs.

Despite an awareness of these data limitations, there has been little improvement in data collection for Native peoples (IOM 2009). The National Congress of American Indians (NCAI), a national advocacy group, the Center for Medicare and Medicaid Services (CMS) Tribal Affairs Group, and the Council of State and Tribal Epidemiologists (CTSE) have all developed policies, statements, and recommendations on improving the collection and reporting of data concerning AIAN populations. These recommendations are summarized as follows:

- *Consult with tribes and communities:* clear and frequent communication to ensure that strategies reflect the priorities of the population, that community support be available, and that communities benefit from improved data; education, outreach, and technical assistance to communities about the research should be provided prior to data collection (Waksberg 2000, NCAI 2010).

- *Improve data collection:* collect hospital discharge data and examine Medicare and Medicaid data, particularly as it pertains to long-term care; collect longitudinal and comprehensive data, including cultural factors; Medicaid, Children's Health Insurance Program (CHIP), and Medicare provider enrollment processes need to identify and keep data on at least three groups of IHS healthcare delivery system providers (Moy et al. 2006, NCAI 2010, OSPE 2007).

- *Reduce racial misclassification:* better collection of data is needed; include NA communities in national data sets and oversample for NA populations (Moy et al. 2006, NCAI 2010).

- *Disaggregate race and ethnicity:* the IOM says that aggregation of race and ethnicity "can mask identification of disparities at the more granular level." The IOM recommends a national scheme should be developed to roll up granular ethnicity categories with locally relevant choices from a standard national list to the applicable broad Office of Management and Budget race and ethnicity categories to the extent feasible (IOM 2009).

- *Standardize categories and consistency:* standardization should be done to enable comparisons across time, location, and settings along with available categorical responses (IOM 2009, NCAI 2010).

- *Coordinate and share across federal agencies:* coordinate and share results of current initiatives that use and collect data on AIANNH health and well-being; integrate IHS data with state hospital discharge data; expand person-based surveys and quality improvement to include Native persons; require Medicaid, CHIP, and Medicare enrollment procedures to identify and keep data; minimize redundancy across agencies (OSPE 2010, Moy et al. 2006, NCAI 2010).

- *Collaborate:* collaboration with states can improve data completeness, accuracy, and consistency. Collaboration with communities and researchers regarding collection and analysis can also help further this goal (OSPE 2010, Moy et al. 2006, CMS Tribal Affairs Group 2010).

- *Perform NA-specific studies*: use existing Medicaid, CHIP, and Medicare enrollment, service use, and payment data; employ quality and effectiveness of care that also examine disparities in treatment and outcomes of care; examine disparities in CMS costs of care for different groups (CMS Tribal Affairs Group 2010).

### Improve Access to Data

Data ownership is a key issue with tribal communities. As discussed in other chapters, in academic institutions it is typically expected that investigators be responsible for the ethical management of the data and publication is a required component of their employment. In addition, US federal agencies assert that since taxpayer dollars fund the projects, the data legally belong to the public and encourage its use and reporting to address multiple concerns. However, acquiring and using health data is often restricted or limited either by tribal nations that assert full ownership or by agencies that invoke rules and regulations such as the Health Insurance Portability and Privacy Act (HIPAA). The HIPAA Privacy Rule is intended to protect the privacy of individually identifiable health information and the HIPAA Security Rule sets national standards for the security of electronic protected health information. The confidentiality provisions of the Patient Safety Rule protect identifiable information being used to analyze and improve patient safety. These rules govern how health data may be collected, used, and reported by whom and to whom. Public health authorities are often reluctant to share health data because of the concerns about violating HIPAA or other privacy laws, thereby limiting access to data to such a degree that a tribe may not be able to get data from the IHS agency that manages their own health clinic.

Tribes and tribal epidemiology centers (TECs) have experienced extensive limitations concerning data sharing with federal, state and local public health authorities. There are 12 TECs across the United States, funded by the IHS and operating in tribal governments, tribal government coalitions (e. g., multitribal health boards) to serve the AIAN population within one of the IHS administrative areas, and urban AIAN populations. TECs provide services in data collection through public health surveillance and epidemiologic research as well as training in public health, response to public health emergencies, provision of technical assistance to tribal communities, and disease control and prevention services. In March 2010, the Indian Health Care Improvement Act (IHCIA) was permanently reauthorized and authorized TECs to be defined and treated as public health authorities specifically to ameliorate problems in data sharing. The reauthorization set in place the authority for TECs to access data, data sets, monitoring systems, delivery systems, and other protected health information through the secretary of the Department of Health and Human Services.

Justifiably, Native Americans are protective of the information that is collected, interpreted, and disseminated and may insist on complete ownership of data. Many communities are interested primarily in public health practice and intervention studies that will provide immediate solutions to health concerns. However, there are hundreds of research studies ongoing in NA communities and the concerns of data collection, management, analysis, and reporting must be addressed. Potential solutions to data stewardship require negotiations between tribal communities, researchers, and funders and may include:

- Creating a data repository in which only specific individuals can access the original data and provide aggregated data to interested outsiders;
- Providing aggregate data rather than raw data; and
- Developing a written contract that sets out specific terms for data sharing.

TECs and other public health entities must seek to have solid working relationships with AIAN communities and be an interested partner in research projects.

### Improve Data Analysis

A saying attributed to former US Surgeon General C. Everett Koop, "Health care is vital to all of us some of the time, but public health is vital to all of us all of the time, (Koop 2003)" is particularly true as many chronic diseases become epidemic in various sectors of the population, and issues such as food safety and food-borne illnesses, flu epidemics, and bacterial infections such as methicillin-resistant *Staphyloccus aureus* (MRSA) infection come to the attention of the general population. Public health has been in existence for well over a hundred years. But because it has not been a topic of interest for the general public, it has received little attention. Usually, when the average person considers public health, he or she thinks of infectious diseases, instead of preventive measures that can be taken to promote healthy lifestyles. Public health is an essential component for the health and safety of populations throughout the world. Public health professionals examine many aspects of prevention from vaccinations to pedestrian paths to increase physical activity as well as environmental health, climate change, emergency preparedness, and antibiotic resistant bacteria (Alliance for Health Reform 2011).

Increased ease of travel among countries provides an avenue for infectious diseases into any country. Many public health professionals question whether the United States as a nation is prepared for potentially deadly viral pandemics. In 2009 WHO declared H1N1 influenza a pandemic worldwide. Increased vaccination against the virus provided protection against further spread, still millions of people in the United States alone were infected, and the potential for other pandemics remains. In a report by the CDC in the *Morbidity and Mortality Weekly Report* (2009) for the AIAN population in 12 states, the H1N1 death rate was four times higher among Native Americans than in all other racial/ethnic populations combined. The reasons are unclear but can likely be attributed to a higher percentage of comorbidities among this population, such as diabetes (45.2%) and asthma (31.0%), that increased the likelihood of complications. This finding is similar to data for other Indigenous populations throughout the world, and is also reflected in data from the 1918–1919 influenza pandemic in which the incidence rate for AIAN persons was three times that of the general population. This includes a 14 to 18 times higher rate in Alaska Natives, a seven times higher rate in Maori individuals, a four times higher rate in Native Hawaiians, and a 4.8 times higher rate in Australian Aboriginals (Mamelund, 2011). Mamelund's research also shows that some of the deaths may have been as much geographical as racial, with more deaths overall in rural communities. Mamelund's data and analysis do not account, however, for the racial disparities in New Zealand and Hawai'i.

Currently, the creation of a public health infrastructure for NA communities in the United States is under development with agencies like the National Indian Health Board (NIHB) and the NCAI assisting NA communities establish and maintain public health infrastructure through education, training, and accreditation. While few tribes have established an accredited public health program, most have programs in place to address public health issues with funds provided on a limited basis through grants and other sources. The Oglala Lakota established tribal ordinances in the 1990s for tribal coroners, fetal alcohol syndrome (FAS) surveillance (personal experience as nurse researcher at the

Aberdeen Area IHS[1] Epidemiology Program, Randall), other public health surveillance and data collection, emergency response to both acute and chronic threats, and to plan, deliver, and evaluate public health at the tribal level. Loretta Bad Heart Bull and Dr. Thomas K. Welty worked with several tribes to put in place ordinances for FAS surveillance during the early 1990s and Dr. Chris Krogh and Leslie L. Randall worked with tribes to establish tribal coroner ordinances on several reservations to allow for better control and faster response to tribal deaths. Tribes were particularly eager to establish these ordinances in order to maintain sovereignty and control what happens within their boundaries regarding health, disease, and death.

The *Healthy People 2020* goals for public health infrastructure include an increase in resources for Native communities to address this area. North Dakota conducted a review of the literature to support putting one of their reservations into one public health unit to offset county health department costs and having the tribe assume more of the costs for healthcare within the borders of the reservation (North Dakota Legislative Council 2011). In 2006, Arizona Governor Janet Napolitano issued an executive order requiring all executive branch agencies to develop and implement tribal consultation policies with tribes in Arizona, designate a member of their staff to assume responsibility for the policy, and review their consultation policies annually. The Maine Legislature established a tribal district composed of lands belonging to the state tribes and any member of a tribe living outside of tribal lands as a Tribal Public Health District Unit for their consultation method; this allows the state to collaborate with and provide public health infrastructure with respect of the people and culture. Through partnerships with federal, state, and local entities and tribes they conduct public health assessment, planning, implementation, and evaluation (North Dakota Legislative Council 2011). As public funds become increasingly scarce, states will examine tribal revenues from gaming and other sources, and there is a strong likelihood that more states will place tribes into their own tribal public health units. As this occurs there will be a need for stronger tribal public health codes and regulations.

---

[1]The Indian Health Service is announcing the name change of the *Aberdeen Area Indian Health Service to the Great Plains Area Indian Health Service* at the request of tribes served by the Aberdeen Area Indian Health Service. See https://federalregister.gov/a/2014-00264 for more information.

In June 2011, the American Public Health Association issued a brief on health workforce provisions called *The Affordable Care Acts Public Health Workforce Provisions: Opportunities and Challenges*. This report gives an overview of the various provisions and what it means for the population. There are few health professionals from minority groups and even fewer AIAN individuals, particularly in public health. From 2008 to 2010 there were approximately 29,000 public health jobs lost at the local departments of health; over 40,000 total were lost by 2011. Budget cuts and personnel cuts were the largest in emergency preparedness divisions, losing 23% of their staff, while the smallest cuts occurred in the divisions of epidemiology and surveillance (9%; NACCHO 2012). Regardless, these contractions mean that prospects for AIAN persons and other minorities to serve in public health are minimal. As a study by Owens et al. (1987) points out, if given a chance at education, NA graduates in public health achieve as much success and have as much satisfaction with their jobs as do their non-Native counterparts. Other studies on the current situation in minority health document that less than 7% of public health staff in executive positions were non-White, and less than 2% were not non-Hispanic White individuals (NACCHO 2012). Of all the local health department personnel, only 0.5% of those were AIAN persons, and 1.9% were NHOPI individuals. It is clear that training, education, and outreach for AIAN persons interested in public health need to occur in order to increase the public health workforce.

## SUMMARY: DATA IS POWER

Native Americans are at elevated risk for many acute and chronic diseases and need the ability to review incidence and prevalence rates in closer detail. Unfortunately, this may not be that easy. Data are not available and, even when accessible, the numbers are often meaningless because data usually cannot be reported at a local or tribal level. This means that tribes and Native communities will need to be more proactive in pursuing research, in involving the community in health-related decisions, and in implementing better data collection, ensuring that those data are relevant to the tribe and the larger Native community. In addition, Native leaders should seek to involve their stakeholders in the research process and in evaluation and intervention strategies designed to improve the health status of their community members.

While many Indigenous people and communities are reluctant to participate in research, many also understand that data collection is a powerful tool for resource advocacy. The problem is that so often the most important information is either incorrect or incomplete. An incorrect or incomplete picture of the health status of a community can negatively influence policy and programming. Dollars, personnel, and other resources are limited, and applying them in the most effective manner is critical to influence the existing disparities and effect positive change. Indigenous communities worldwide and multinational groups are working to improve the quality of the data that describe Indigenous communities. The US National Center for Health Statistics leads a collaboration with colleagues from Canada, Australia, and New Zealand to improve and report morbidity and mortality data on Native populations. The University of Hawai'i at Manoa is leading the effort to develop an Indigenous health degree program with colleagues from Australia, Canada, New Zealand, and the Native American Research and Training Center at the University of Arizona. Developing a critical mass of "data warriors" and Indigenous scientists is critical to eradicate the problems that continue to plague Indigenous people despite advances in medicine and public health.

Finally, we cannot attribute disparities in health and well-being solely to risk factors or race/ethnicity and mask the effects of socioeconomic disadvantage that are inter-related and connected to colonization (Reading 2010, Beauchamp et al. 2004, Carson et al. 2007, Health Canada 2003, Reading et al. 2007). Policies and programs that counter such effects are not only needed but also owed to the first peoples of North America.

## REFERENCES

Administration for Children and Families, Office of Child Care. 2012. *Fiscal Years 2010 and 2011 Tribal Home Visiting Grantees & Abstracts.* Available at: http://www.acf.hhs. gov/programs/occ/resource/affordable-care-act-tribal-maternal-infant-and-early-childhood-home. Accessed March 23, 2012.

Alliance for Health Reform. 2011. *Health Care Workforce: Future Supply vs Demand.* Available at: http://healthinfo.montana.edu/MTHWAC/Health_Care_Workforce_104. pdf. Accessed June 16, 2011.

American Public Health Association. 2011. *The Affordable Care Act's Public Health Workforce Provisions: Opportunities and Challenges. Community Transformation*

*Grants (Section 4201)*. Available at: http://www.ncsl.org/issues-research/health/affordable-care-act-grants-awarded-to-states.aspx. Accessed March 23, 2012.

Asian and Pacific Islander Health Forum. 2010. *Native Hawaiian and Pacific Islander Health Disparities*. Available at: http://www.apiahf.org/sites/default/files/NHPI_Report08a_2010.pdf. Accessed June 10, 2013.

Assembly of First Nations/First Nations Information Governance Committee. 2007. *The First Nations Regional Longitudinal Health Survey (RHS), 2002/03*. 2nd edition. Available at: http://www.rhs-ers.ca. Accessed May 28, 2013.

Barnes P, Adams P, Powell-Griner E. 2005. Health characteristics of the American Indian and Alaska Native adult population: United States, 1999–2003. *Advance Data From Vital and Health Statistics*. Hyattsville, MD: National Center for Health Statistics. 356:1–24.

Beals J, Novins D, Whitesell N, et al. 2005. Prevalence of mental disorders and utilization of mental health services in two American Indian reservation populations: Mental health disparities in a national context. *Am J Psych*. 162:1723–1732.

Beauchamp J, Blaauwbroek M, Brulé C, et al. 2004. *Improving the Health of Canadians*. Ottawa, ON: Canadian Institute of Health Information.

Beavis MA, Klos N, Carter T, et al. 1997. *Literature Review: Aboriginal Peoples and Homelessness*. Ottawa, ON: Canada Mortgage and Housing Corporation.

Berry M, Reynoso C, Braceras J, et al. 2004. *Broken Promises: Evaluating the Native American Health Care System*. Washington, DC: US Commission on Civil Rights.

Bliss A, Cobb N, Solomon T, et al. 2008. Lung cancer incidence among American Indians and Alaska Natives in the United States, 1999–2004. *Cancer Suppl*. 113(5):168–1178.

Bobet E. 1997. *Diabetes among First Nations People: Information from the 1991 Aboriginal Peoples Survey carried out by Statistics Canada* (Report). Ottawa, ON: Medical Services Branch, Health Canada.

Booth H. 1999. Pacific island suicide in comparative perspective. *J Biosoc Sci*. 31, 433–448.

Carson B, Dunbar T, Chenhall RD, et al. 2007. *Social Determinants of Indigenous Health*. Crows Nest, Australia: Allen & Unwin.

Castor ML, Smyser MS, Taualii MM, et al. 2006. A nationwide population-based study identifying health disparities between American Indians/Alaska Natives and the general populations living in select urban counties. *Am J Public Health.* 96(8):1478–1484.

Center on the Family. 2012. *Homeless Service Utilization Report.* Available at: http:// uhfamily.hawaii.edu/publications/brochures/HomelessServiceUtilization2012.pdf. Accessed June 11, 2013.

Center for Medicaid and Medicare Services Tribal Affairs Group. 2010. *American Indian and Alaska Native Data Symposium: Developing Medicaid and Medicare Data Summary of the Proceedings.* Available at: http://www.edfoxphd.com/Data_Symposium _report_9_27_10-5_copy.pdf. Accessed June 16, 2013.

Centers for Disease Control and Prevention. 2009. Alcohol and suicide among racial/ethnic populations – 17 states, 2005–2006. *MMWR Morb Mortal Wkly Rep.* 58(23):637–641.

Centers for Disease Control and Prevention. 2009. Youth risk behavior surveillance system, United States 2009. *MMWR Morb Mortal Wkly Rep.* 57(SS-5):1–148.

Centers for Disease Control and Prevention. 2011. Youth online: High school YRBS 2011 results. Available at: http://apps.nccd.cdc.gov/youthonline/App/Default.aspx?SID= HS. Accessed December 10, 2013.

Centers for Disease Control and Prevention. 2009. Deaths related to 2009 H1N1 influenza among American Indian/Alaska Natives (AIANs)-12 states, 2009. *MMWR Morb Mortal Wkly Rep.* 58(48):1341–1344.

Centers for Disease Control and Prevention, National Center for HIV/AIDS, Viral Hepatitis, STD, and TB Prevention. *Epidemiologic Profile 2010: Asians and Native Hawaiians and Other Pacific Islanders.* Atlanta, GA: Centers for Disease Control and Prevention. 2012: [53–59].

Centers for Disease Control and Prevention. 2012. *Deaths: Final Data for 2009. National Vital Statistics Reports 60(03): Tables 16 and 17.* Available at: http://www.cdc. gov/nchs/data/nvsr/nvsr60/nvsr60_03.pdf. Accessed July 12, 2013.

Centers for Disease Control and Prevention. 2013. *HIV Surveillance Report, 2011 v23.* Available at: http://www.cdc.gov/hiv/topics/surveillance/resources/reports. Accessed June 10, 2013.

Centers for Disease Control and Prevention, Indian Health Service. 2009. *Indian Health Surveillance Report: Sexually Transmitted Diseases, 2007.* Available at: http://www.cdc. gov/std/stats/ihs/ihs-survrpt_web508nov2009.pdf. Accessed July 12, 2013.

Centers for Disease Control and Prevention, National Center for Health Statistics. 2011. *Compressed Mortality File 1999–2008 2012b. CDC WONDER On-line Database, compiled from Multiple Cause of Death File 2008, Series 20 No. 2M, 2011.* Available at: http://wonder.cdc.gov/ucd-icd10.html. Accessed January 10, 2012.

Centers for Disease Control and Prevention, National Center for Health Statistics. Health, United States, 2007. Table 19. Available at: http://www.cdc.gov/nchs/data/hus/ hus07.pdf. Accessed November 1, 2013.

Centers for Disease Control and Prevention, National Center for HIV/AIDS, Viral Hepatitis, STD, and TB Prevention. 2012. *Epidemiologic Profile 2010: Asians and Native Hawaiians and Other Pacific Islanders.* Available at: http://www.cdc.gov/nchhstp/ publications/docs/AsianNativeHawaiianEpiProfileReport-20120727.pdf. Accessed July 12, 2013.

Centers for Disease Control, Office of Minority Health. 2009. *10 Leading Causes of Death: Native Hawaiian and Other Pacific Island Populations.* Available at: http://www. cdc.gov/minorityhealth/populations/REMP/nhopi.html#. Accessed June 10, 2013.

Chiem B, Nguyen V, Wu PL, et al. 2006. Cardiovascular risk factors among Chamorros. *BMC Public Health.* Dec 8;6:298.

City and County of Honolulu. 2012. *Homeless Point in Time Count.* Available at: http:// www.hawaiihomeless.org/Links_files/Oahu%20PIT%20Report%202012%20FINAL.pdf. Accessed June 11, 2013.

Collins VR, Dowse GK, Toelupe PM, et al. 1994. Increasing prevalence of NIDDM in the Pacific Island population of Western Samoa over a 13-year period. *Diabetes Care.* 17(4):288–296.

Daniel M, Gamble D, Henderson J, et al. 1995. Diabetes prevalence, behavioural and anthropometric risk factors, and psychosocial constructs in three Aboriginal communities in central British Columbia. *Chronic Dis Can.* 16(4).

Dappleton Research Team. 2003. *GVRD Aboriginal Homelessness Study 2003 (Abridged).* Available at: http://chodarr.org/sites/default/files/chodarr1483.pdf. Accessed July 12, 2013.

Delisle HF, Rivard M, Ekoe JM. 1995. Prevalence estimates of diabetes and of other cardiovascular risk factors in the two largest Algonquin communities of Quebec. *Diabetes Care.* 18(9):1255–1259.

EagleStaff ML, Klug MG, Burd L. 2006. Infant mortality reviews in the Aberdeen Area of the Indian Health Service: strategies and outcomes. *Public Health Rep.* 121(2):140–148.

Eaglestaff M, Klug MG, Burd L. 2007. Eight years of infant mortality reviews in the Aberdeen Area of the Indian Health Service. *IHS Provider.* June:174–180.

Else IRN, Andrade NN, Nahulu LB. 2007. Suicide and suicidal-related behaviors among indigenous Pacific islanders in the United States. *Death Studies.* 31:479–501.

First Nations Centre. 2005. *First Nations Regional Longitudinal Health Survey (RHS) 2002/2003: Results for Adults, Youth and Children Living in First Nations Communities.* Ottawa, ON: First Nations Centre at the National Aboriginal Health Organization.

First Nations Centre. 2007. *First Nations Regional Longitudinal Health Survey (RHS) 2002/2003 Rev. The Peoples Report.* 2nd edition. Available at: http://www.rhs-ers.ca/ sites/default/files/ENpdf/RHS_2002/rhs2002-03-the_peoples_report_afn.pdf. Accessed June 5, 2013.

First Nations Centre. 2007. *First Nations Regional Longitudinal Health Survey (RHS) Phase 1 (2002/2003) Quick Facts.* Available at: http://www.rhs-ers.ca. Accessed June 5, 2013.

Folsom DP, Hawthorne W, Lindamer L, et al. 2005. Prevalence and risk factors for homelessness and utilization of mental health services among 10,340 patients with serious mental illness in a large public mental health system. *Am J Psych.* 162:370–376.

Gavin L, MacKay AP, Brown K, et al. 2009. Sexual and reproductive health of persons aged 10–24 years—United States, 2002–2007. *MMWR CDC Surveill Summ.* 58(6):1–58.

Goldsmith SK, Pellmar TC, Kleinman AM, Bunney WE, editors. 2002. *Reducing Suicide: A National Imperative.* Washington, DC: National Academy Press.

Grandinetti A, Chang HK, Mau MK, et al. 1998. Prevalence of glucose intolerance among native Hawaiians in two rural communities. *Diabetes Care.* 21(4): 549–554.

Hawai'i State Department of Health. 2007. *The Burden of Cardiovascular Disease in Hawai'i 2007.* Available at: http://hawaii.gov/health/statistics/brfss/reports/CVDBurden_Rpt2007.pdf. Accessed July 12, 2013.

Hawai'i H.O.M.E. Project. 2009. *Homeless in Hawaii.* Available at: http://www.hawaiihomeproject.org/homelesshawaii.html. Accessed June 11, 2013.

Hawai'i Interagency Council on Homelessness. 2008. *Plan to End Homelessness in Hawai'i.* Rev. Sept. 2008. Available at: http://www.hawaiihomeless.org/Home_files/10%20year%20Plan-HI%20rev%200908.pdf. Accessed September 11, 2013.

Health Canada. 2003. *The Statistical Profile on Health of First Nations in Canada. Vital Statistics for Atlantic and Western Canada, 2001/2002.* Available at: http://www.hc-sc.gc.ca/fniah-spnia/pubs/aborig-autoch/stats-profil-atlant/index-eng.php. Accessed June 11, 2013.

Health Canada. 2003. *Arthritis in Canada. An Ongoing Challenge.* Available at: http://www.phac-aspc.gc.ca/publicat/ac. Accessed June 10, 2013.

Health Canada. 2005. *A Statistical Profile on the Health of First Nations in Canada for the Year 2000.* Ottawa, ON: Health Canada.

Health Canada. 2009. *A Statistical Profile on the Health of First Nations in Canada: Self-Rated Health and Selected Conditions, 2002–2005.* Ottawa, ON: Health Canada.

Health Canada. 2012. *First Nations and Inuit Health: HIV and AIDS.* Available at: http://www.hc-sc.gc.ca/fniah-spnia/diseases-maladies/aids-sida/index-eng.php. Accessed June 10, 2013.

Health Canada. 2013. *Canadian Alcohol and Drug Use Monitoring Survey (CADUMS) 2011.* Available at: http://www.hc-sc.gc.ca/hc-ps/drugs-drogues/stat/_2011/summary-sommaire-eng.php. Accessed June 10, 2013.

Health Research Services Agency. 2010. *Health Center Program: Special Populations Primary Health Care: Health Center Program.* Available at: http://bphc.hrsa.gov/about/specialpopulations. Accessed November 1, 2013.

Helin S. 2002. *Aboriginal Homelessness, Prince Rupert and Port Edward: An Assets and Gap Review of Existing Services for the Homeless.* Prince Rupert, British Columbia: Prince Rupert Steering Committee on Aboriginal Homelessness.

Hellerstedt WL, Peterson-Hickey M, Rhodes KL, et al. 2006. Environmental, social, and personal correlates of having ever had sexual intercourse among American Indian youths. *Am J Public Health.* 96(12):2228-2234.

Heron MP, Smith BL. 2007. Deaths: leading causes for 2003. *National Vital Statistics Reports.* vol 55 no 10. Hyattsville, MD: National Center for Health Statistics. Available at: http://www.cdc.gov/nchs/data/nvsr/nvsr55/nvsr55_10.pdf. Accessed July 12, 2013.

Hixson L, Hepler B, Kim MO. 2012. *The Native Hawaiian and Other Pacific Islander Population: 2010. Census Briefs.* Available at: http://www.census.gov/prod/cen2010/briefs/c2010br-12.pdf. Accessed May 28, 2013.

Holman RC, Curns AT, Kaufman SF, et al. 2001. Trends in infectious disease hospitalizations among American Indians and Alaska Natives. *Am J Public Health.* 91(3):425-31.

Hwang SW. 2001. Homelessness and health. *CMAJ (Ottawa).* 164(2):229-233.

Indian Health Service. 2002. *Regional Differences in Indian Health (2000-2001).* Available at: http://www.ihs.gov/NonMedicalPrograms/IHS%5Fsta ts/IHS_HQ_Publications.asp. Accessed November 3, 2005.

Indian Health Service. 2013. *Indian Health Disparities.* Available at: http://www.ihs.gov/newsroom/includes/themes/newihstheme/display_objects/documents/factsheets/Disparities_2013.pdf. Accessed March 1, 2013.

Institute of Medicine. 2009. *Toward Health Equity and Patient-Centeredness: Integrating Health Literacy, Disparities Reduction, and Quality Improvement: Workshop Summary.* Washington, DC: The National Academies Press.

Janz T, Seto J, Turner A. 2009. *Aboriginal Peoples Survey, 2006. An Overview of the Health of the Métis Population.* Ottawa, ON: Statistics Canada.

Kliewer E, Mayer T, Wajda A. 2002. *The Health of Manitoba's Métis Population and their Utilization of Medical Services: A Pilot Study.* Winnipeg, MB: CancerCare Manitoba and Manitoba Health.

Karch DL, Logan J, McDaniel D, et al. 2012. Surveillance for violent deaths—National Violent Death Reporting System, 16 states, 2009. *MMWR Surveill Summ.* 61:1-43. Available at: http://www.cdc.gov/mmwr/preview/mmwrhtml/ss6106a1.htm?s_cid=ss6106a1_e#tab6. Accessed February 13, 2011.

Kasprow WJ, Rosenheck RA. 1998. Substance use and psychiatric problems of homeless Native American veterans. *Psychiatr Serv.* 49(3):345–50.

Kaufman CE, Desserich J, Big Crow CK, et al. 2007. Culture, context, and sexual risk among Northern Plains American Indian youth. *Soc Sci Med.* 64:2152–2164.

Koop CE. 2003, Association of Schools of Public Health MD, former US Surgeon General (Association of Schools of Public Health, 2003).

Lee KK. 2000. Urban Poverty in Canada: A Statistical Profile. Available at: http://www.ccsd.ca/pubs/2000/up. Accessed July 13, 2013.

Luo ZC, Kierans WJ, Wilkins R, et al. 2004a. Infant mortality among first nations versus non-first nations in British Columbia: temporal trends in rural versus urban areas, 1981–2000. *Int J Epidemiol.* 33(6):1252–9.

Luo ZC, Wilkins R, Heaman M, et al. 2010b. Neighbourhood socio- economic characteristics, birth outcomes and infant mortality among First Nations and non-First Nations in Manitoba, Canada. *Open Womens Health J.* 4:55–61.

Luo ZC, Wilkins R, Platt RW, et al. 2004b. Risks of adverse pregnancy outcomes among Inuit and North American Indian women in Quebec, 1985–97. *Paediatr Perinat Epidemiol.* 18(1):40–50.

Magin JL. December 5, 2006. Hawaii's burgeoning homeless population seeks refuge on. *The New York Times.* Available at: http://www.nytimes.com/2006/12/05/world/americas/05iht-hawaii.3784081.html. Accessed July 13, 2013.

Mamelund SE. 2011. Geography may explain adult mortality from the 1918–20 influenza pandemic. *Epidemics.* 3(1):46–60.

Martin JA, Hamilton BE, Sutton PD, et al. 2010. *Births: Final Data for 2007. National Vital Statistics Reports.* Vol. 58, No. 24. Hyattsville, MD: National Center for Health Statistics.

Mathews TJ, MacDorman MF. 2012. *Infant Mortality Statistics From the 2009 Period Linked Birth/Infant Death Data Set. National Vital Statistics Reports.* Vol. 61, No. 8. Hyattsville, MD: National Center for Health Statistics.

McBean AM. 2006. Improving Medicare's data on race and ethnicity. *Medicare Brief.* Oct(15): 1–7.

Meade CS, Ickovics JR. 2005. Systematic review of sexual risk among pregnant and mothering teens in the USA: pregnancy as an opportunity for integrated prevention of STD and repeat pregnancy. *Soc Sci Med.* 60(4):661–78.

Miller B, Chu KC, Hankey BF, et al. 2008. Cancer incidence and mortality patterns among specific Asian and Pacific Islander populations in the US Cancer Causes Control. 2008. 19(3): 227-256.

Moy E, Smith CR, Johansson P, et al. 2006. Gaps in data for American Indians and Alaska Natives in the National Healthcare Disparities Report. *Am Indian Alsk Native Mental Health Res.* 13(1):52–69.

National Association of County & City Health Officials. 2012. *Local Health Department Job Losses and Program Cuts: Findings From January 2012 Survey.* Available at: http://www.naccho.org/advocacy/resources/upload/LHD-Budget-Cuts-two-pager.pdf. March 25, 2012.

National Campaign to Prevent Teen and Unplanned Pregnancy. 2008. *American Indian/Alaska Native Youth and Teen Pregnancy Prevention.* Available at: http://www.thenationalcampaign.org/resources/sciencesays.aspx. Accessed July 16, 2011.

National Center for Health Statistics. 2011. *Health, United States, 2010: With Special Feature on Death and Dying.* Hyattsville, MD: National Center for Health Statistics.

National Congress of American Indians. 2010. *Data Collection.* Available at: http://files.ncai.org/ncai_events/2010_WH_Summit/1j_-_Data_Collection_-_FINAL.pdf. Accessed July 13, 2013.

North Dakota Legislative Council. 2011. *October Minutes.* Available at: http://www.legis.nd.gov/assembly/62-2011. Accessed March 22, 2013.

Office of the Assistant Secretary for Planning and Evaluation. 2007. *Gaps and Strategies for Improving AI/AN/NA Data: Final Report.* Available at: http://aspe.hhs.gov/hsp/07/AI-AN-NA-data-gaps. Accessed July 13, 2013.

Office Of Hawaiian Affairs. OHA Public Information Office. 2006. OHA joins governor's effort to find solutions and relief to widespread homelessness on Oahu's Leeward Coast. Available at: http://www.highbeam.com/doc/1P3-1091364001.html. Accessed September 29, 2013.

Okihiro M, Harrigan R. 2005. An overview of obesity and diabetes in the diverse populations of the Pacific. *Ethn Dis.* 15(suppl 5):471–80.

Ontario Federation of Indian Friendship Centres. 2004. *Urban Aboriginal Child Poverty Background*. Available at: http://www.ofifc.org/ofifchome/page/notes.htm. Accessed July 8, 2008.

Owens MV, Cameron CM, Hickman P. 1987. Job achievements of Indian and non-Indian graduates in public health: how do they compare? *Public Health Rep.* 102(4):372–376.

Panapasa SV, Mau MK, Williams DR, et al. 2010. Mortality patterns of Native Hawaiians across their lifespan: 1990–2000. *Am J Public Health.* 100(11): 2304–2310.

Perez R. October 21, 2006. Health neglect strains main medical facility. Honolulu Advertiser. Available at: http://the.honoluluadvertiser.com/article/2006/Oct/21/ln/FP610210347.html. Accessed January 5, 2010.

Public Health Agency of Canada. 2009. *Summary: Estimates of HIV Prevalence and Incidence in Canada, 2008.* Available at: http://www.phac-aspc.gc.ca/aids-sida/publication/survreport/estimat08-eng.php. Accessed December 1, 2009.

Public Health Agency of Canada. 2007. *HIV/AIDS Epi Updates, November 2007.* Available at: http://www.phac-aspc.gc.ca/aids-sida/publication/epi/pdf/epi2007_e.pdf. Accessed November 1, 2009.

Reading J. 2010. *The Crisis of Chronic Disease among Aboriginal Peoples: A Challenge for Public Health, Population Health and Society.* Victoria, BC: University of Victoria Centre for Aboriginal Health Research.

Reading J, Kmetic A, Gideon V. 2007. First nations wholistic policy and planning model. AFN discussion paper for the World Health Organization Commission on Social Determinants of Health. Ottawa, ON: Assembly of First Nations.

Ring I, Brown N. 2003. The health status of indigenous peoples and others. *BMJ.* 327(7412): 404–405.

Rutman S, Park A, Castor M, et al. 2008. Urban American Indian and Alaska Native youth: Youth risk behavior survey 1997–2003. *Matern Child Health J.* 12(1):76–81.

Sloan NR. 1963. Ethnic distribution of diabetes mellitus in Hawaii. *JAMA.* 183(6):419–424.

Smylie J, Crengle S, Freemantle J, et al. 2010. Indigenous birth outcomes in Australia, Canada, New Zealand and the United States – an overview. *Open Womens Health J.* 2010(4):1–11.

Smylie J, Fell D, Ohlsson A, et al. 2010. A review of Aboriginal infant mortality rates in Canada: striking and persistent Aboriginal/non-Aboriginal inequities. *Can J Public Health.* 101(2):143–148.

Statistics Canada. 2003. *National Longitudinal Survey of Children and Youth, Cycle 4 2000/2001.* Available at: http://www23.statcan.gc.ca/imdb/p2SV.pl?Function= getSurvey&SurvId=4450&SurvVer=1&InstaId=16044&InstaVer=4&SDDS= 4450&lang=en&db=imdb&adm=8&dis=2. Accessed July 13, 2013.

Statistics Canada. 2008a. *Aboriginal Children's Survey, 2006: Family, Community and Child Care.* Ottawa, ON: Statistics Canada.

Statistics Canada. 2008b. *Aboriginal Peoples in Canada in 2006: Inuit, Métis and First Nations, 2006 Census.* Ottawa, ON: Statistics Canada.

Khandour E, Mason K. 2007. *Street Health Report 2007: Highlights and Action Plan.* Available at: http://www.streethealth.ca/downloads/the-street-health-report-2007-highlights-action-plan.pdf. Accessed July 13, 2013.

Substance Abuse and Mental Health Services Administrations. 2010. *Substance Use Among American Indian or Alaska Native Adults. National Survey on Drug Use and Health.* Available at: http://www.oas.samhsa.gov/2k10/182/AmericanIndian.htm. Accessed June 15, 2013.

Suicide Prevention Resource Center. 2009. *Hawaii Suicide Prevention Fact Sheet: Suicides, 1999–2005.Summary Health Statistics for US Adults: 2008. Table 6.* Available at: http://www.cdc.gov/nchs/data/series/sr_10/sr10_242.pdf. July 13, 2013.

Tjepkema M. 2002. *The Health of the Off-Reserve Aboriginal Population.* Ottawa, ON: Statistics Canada.

United States Conference of Mayors – Sodexho, Inc. 2006. *Hunger and Homelessness Survey: A Status Report on Hunger and Homelessness in America's Cities.* Available at: http://usmayors.org/hungersurvey/2006/report06.pdf. Accessed July 13, 2013.

Urban Indian Health Institute, Seattle Indian Health Board. 2009. *Visibility Through Data: Health Information for Urban American Indian and Alaska Native Communities.* Seattle, WA: Urban Indian Health Institute.

Waksberg J, Levine D, Marker D. 2000. *Assessment of Major Federal Data Sets for Analyses of Hispanic and Asian or Pacific Islander Subgroups and Native Americans: Task 3 Report: Extending the Utility of Federal Databases.* Rockville, MD: Westat.

Weisman JS, Hasnain-Wynia R. 2011. Advancing health care equity through improved data collection. *N Engl J Med.* 364:2276–2277.

Wente M. 2000. *Urban Aboriginal Homelessness in Canada.* Toronto, ON: University of Toronto.

Wingo PA, Lesesne CA, Smith RA, et al. 2011. Geographic variation in trends and characteristics of teen childbearing among American Indians and Alaska Natives, 1990–2007. *Matern Child Health J.* 16(9):1779–1790.

Yamane DP, Oeser SG, Omori J. 2010. Health disparities in the Native Hawaiian homeless. *Hawaii Med J.* 69(Suppl 3):635–41.

World Health Organization Commission on Social Determinants of Health. 2007. *Social Determinants of Indigenous Health: The International Experience and its Policy Implications.* Adelaide, Australia: Finders University.

Yuen NY, Nahulu LB, Hishinuma ES, et al. 2000. Cultural identification and attempted suicide in Native Hawaiian adolescents. *J Am Acad Child Adolesc Psychiatry.* 39(3):360–367.

Yusuf S, Reddy S, Ounpuu S, et al. 2001. Global burden of cardiovascular diseases: Part II: variations in cardiovascular disease by specific ethnic groups and geographic regions and prevention strategies. *Circulation.* 104(23):2855–2864.

Zerger S. 2004. *Health Care for Homeless Native Americans.* Available at: http://www.turtleisland.org/healing/homeless.pdf. Accessed July 13, 2013.

# 3

# Building Relationships: Step One for Researchers Working With Indian Communities

Leslie L. Randall, RN, MPH, BSN

## INTRODUCTION

This chapter covers the basics of building a research relationship with American Indian and Alaska Native (AIAN) communities for both the researcher and the tribal community. The discussion includes a background on institutional review boards (IRBs); discussion of tribal communication strategies; issues related to data, data management, and data ownership; and the implications of conducting research in tribal communities. This discussion will focus on reservation communities; for information and discussion of this issue as it pertains to urban Indian communities, the author suggests reviewing the report *Urban Indian Health* by Fouquera (2001).

"Research" is frequently considered a dirty word in Indigenous communities (Pyett 2002, Smith 1999). The following discussion focuses on how to overcome this perspective within tribal communities by establishing mutually productive collaborative relationships with tribes. The examples illustrate the intricacies of working with tribal communities and provide an introduction for the chapters that follow. Working with tribal communities is especially important because funding agencies are increasingly incorporating collaborative or participatory research requirements into their application process.

## FIRST STEPS AND COLLABORATION

Community involvement is a necessary component of research conducted with tribes. IRBs are conditioned to examine research with a view to minimizing risk to the individual, but with the smaller communities that represent AIAN research, a different standard is essential to ensure that the risk to the community and the individual are addressed (American Academy of Pediatrics Committee on Native American Child Health 2004, Kaufert et al. 1999). For example, it is often possible to identify an individual of a small community, even if not examining a relatively rare disease, simply from demographic information. In addition, the uniqueness derived from their cultural differences, language, customs, and area of residence can serve as identifiers for small tribes or tribal communities. As Manson et al. (2004) note, the consequences of conducting research in AIAN communities without the collaboration and input of the specific community range from stigmatization to economic harm, but collaboration with tribes minimizes these risks. The economic effect can range from loss of funding for programs to loss of insurance for the individual or family through genetic identification of risk (Pyett 2002, American Academy of Pediatrics Committee on Native American Child Health 2004, Kaufert et al. 1999, Manson et al. 2004, Dukepoo 1998).

Other risks to the community or an identified participant are social, legal, or political. Social risk involves stigmatization of the individual or community, resulting in scientific racism (Sharp and Foster 2002). An example of this type of social risk is the stigmatization of AIAN persons and alcohol through the stereotype of the drunken Indian and the related perception that fetal alcohol syndrome disorders occur only in AIAN populations. An example of political risk is the controversy surrounding the Kennewick Man, in which the accepted history of the AIAN community as the original inhabitants of this continent is being questioned (American Academy of Pediatrics Committee on Native American Child Health 2004, Manson et al. 2004, Sharp and Foster 2002). In 1996, part of a human skull was found on the bottom of the Columbia River in Kennewick, Washington; later searches of the area turned up a nearly complete male skeleton. The remains were labeled "Kennewick Man" or the "Ancient One" and identified as being between 8,000 and 9,500 years old, one of the oldest and most complete skeletons found in North America. He became the subject of a lawsuit between the federal government with Native American tribes, as there were disputes over the handling of the bones, the burial of the discovery site, and statements by some scholars that suggested the skeleton was Caucasian, thus implying that Europeans may have reached the Americas before Indians did (Davis 2004, Powell et al. 1999). This example is typical of the kinds of miscommunication that occur when two cultures interact and that each tribe faces when dealing with the outside. Whether the Ancient One was Caucasian or American Indian is not the point for tribal people; what is important to tribal people is that the Ancient One was obviously a part of the culture during that era and that he was buried intact (Davis 2004, Powell et al. 1999). He is therefore an "ancestor." This controversy over the Ancient One highlights the need to understand the hostility that often accompanies misconceptions, miscommunications, ideologies, and beliefs related to what it means to be American Indian and Alaska Native. So many efforts by the US government continue to focus on the goal of total assimilation of the tribes even though the government promotes self-governance and self-determination. Laws and policies often contradict this, as noted by Bruyneel (2007):

> In the contemporary era, American political actors, organizations, governments, and institutions, such as Arnold Schwarzenegger, CERA[1], the city of Sherrill[2], and the US Supreme Court, have come to see Indigenous tribes as too strong to be recognized as sovereign governments. This contrasts with the situation in the late nineteenth century, when Americans generally viewed Indigenous tribes as too weak to be recognized as sovereign governments. What this means for contemporary US–Indigenous relations is that on top of engaging in a postcolonial resistance against American colonial impositions, another of the many tasks for Indigenous political actors is to articulate how the expression of political power by Indigenous tribes and citizens is more often than not a supplementary strategy rather than one by which Indigenous people seek either to be assimilated within or to displace the liberal democratic settler-state and nation.

As noted in the preceding quote, maintaining tribal sovereignty is an important issue for tribal communities and ensuring that anyone who comes into the community understands this is paramount. Communicating with the

---

[1] Citizens Equal Rights Alliance.

[2] US Supreme Court decision in *City of Sherrill, New York v. Oneida Nation of New York (2005)*.

tribal community regarding the research becomes a means of acknowledging that sovereignty and helps to maintain good relationships. Methods of minimizing the risk of miscommunication include engaging the tribes in the development of the research proposal, learning the community issues, and exploring ways to involve tribes with research efforts (Kaufert et al. 1999, Manson et al. 2004). These methods are important to ensure the participation of tribes and tribal communities in the research process and avoiding or minimizing risk to the AIAN community.

However, these steps are only the beginning of the process. The success of the research and continued involvement of the community require the researcher to communicate with community members, include tribal members as co-investigators, and hire and train local community staff. Tribal elders, community members, the tribal council, elected tribal officials, tribal health directors, trusted researchers, local health professionals, spiritual or religious organizations, traditional or spiritual leaders, and women are some of the stakeholders whose input is necessary to the development of the research proposal or agenda. Each stakeholder plays a role in the community that can be important to the development of the research project. Tribal elders provide a unique perspective of tribal history, culture, wisdom, and memory (Clarke 1991). Elder status is attained through a variety of means: being the oldest in the family, personal standing in the community, religious standing, and age. As the authors of the Swinomish Tribal Mental Health Project point out, "Elders are the teachers and carriers of tradition" (Clarke 1991, p. 154). Community members understand the environment, culture, and social context.

Tribal councils and elected members represent the rest of the community and have the power to approve and support the research. Other trusted researchers carry institutional memory of issues and experiences within the community that are essential for success. Local health professionals are familiar with the health problems in the community and can provide anecdotal information about the community. Spiritual or religious organizations and leaders provide information on what is and is not acceptable within the context of religious or spiritual beliefs within the community. Finally, women are considered the core of the AIAN community, wielding a fundamental influence within the community. As Medicine points out in *Encyclopedia of North American Indians –Women:*

Indian women are often seen as culture brokers as well as the primary transmitters of Indigenous culture. As a consequence, Indian women—often assisted by men—have maintained the mechanisms both for adaptation and for encouraging the continuity of traditional cultures in the modern age (1996).

## INSTITUTIONAL REVIEW BOARDS

This section will discuss the tribes within the IHS health care system, which serves only those tribes that are federally recognized. In addition to consultation, approvals are needed. These approvals include, but are not limited to, tribal council approval, Indian Health Service (IHS) IRB approval, and director or CEO approval when IHS data, staff, or facilities are involved. Some tribes have internal research committees and IRBs that also need to be approached for approval. Since each tribe covered under the IHS IRB is considered a sovereign nation either under treaty or by federal recognition, tribes have the power to approve or disapprove research within their jurisdiction (Kickingbird 2000). The approval process involves requesting a written resolution or letter of support from the tribe or from their recognized representative, such as the Northwest Portland Area Indian Health Board (NPAIHB) for tribes in the Northwest Area (Oregon, Idaho, and Washington) or Great Plains Tribal Chairmen's Health Board (formerly the Aberdeen Area Tribal Chairmen's Health Board, or AATCHB) for tribes in the Dakotas, Iowa, and Nebraska. The IHS is divided into 12 areas with specific states assigned in each area (Figure 3.1). Most areas have an IRB, which operates under the umbrella of the national IHS IRB. As an increasing number of tribes develop their own IRBs, such as in the Navajo Area (Navajo serves as both the area IRB and the tribal IRB) and the Alaska Area under 45 Code of Federal Regulations (CFR) 46. As such, researchers should become familiar with the tribal IRB process. If the research is to take place in an IHS-funded clinic or hospital, the approval of the area IRB or the national IRB (or sometimes both) is required before implementing a research study. If the research takes place in a tribally compacted facility (see discussion in Chapter 1) only the tribal IRB or tribal council (depending upon the tribe) approval is required. If it is a tribal research program (which is not covered under 45 CFR 46) that approves the research, it still needs IHS or tribal IRB approval.

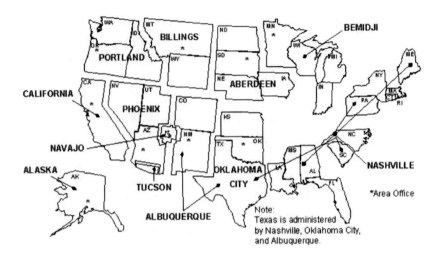

**Figure 3.1. Indian Health Service Area Offices.**
*Source:* Regional Differences in Indian Health 2002-2003.

IRBs strive to examine each protocol based on the following three criteria: (1) respect for persons, (2) beneficence (to do no harm and to maximize benefit), and (3) justice (Kickingbird 2000). Each IHS IRB adds the fourth criterion of *protection of the community as a whole* and endeavors to ensure that there is informed consent, which accurately describes benefits and risks to both the individual and the community. Protection of the whole community is an important aspect of the review process for IHS IRBs, and this is where they differ from other IRBs (IHS 2009). As the previous IHS Director of Research, Dr. Phillip L. Smith, said it best:

> Of all the things that I think when I work with the tribes I tell them they have the ultimate authority. Research as a whole is usually elective. You don't need to do it. It is a good thing to do it. It is the right thing to do, but it is elective. And you could always say no.

The name and address of each IHS Area IRB chair can be found on the IHS Research Program Web site (http://www.ihs.gov/MedicalPrograms/Research/index.cfm). Every IHS IRB reviews each protocol according to 45 CFR Part 46, *Protection of Human Subjects* (US Department of Health and Human Services 2009). The national IHS IRB and area IRB often simultaneously review research protocols. Because of the time lag that may be involved, the researcher should submit the proposal to both IRBs at the same time, especially if the research involves more than minimal risk. The national IRB checks with the area IRB to ensure that both have copies of the proposal. The national IRB requires that the area IRB approve the protocol first, and if the protocol is of minimal risk to human participants the national IRB will likely defer to the area IRB. Most area IRBs require the researcher to submit the proposal to them a minimum of two weeks prior to formal review, to allow researchers time to communicate with IRB chairs regarding the completeness and accuracy of one's research protocol. One of the main obstacles to getting the protocol approved is lacking all the approvals from the tribal stakeholders in place. For guidelines on the IRB submission process, refer to the Northwest Portland Area Indian Health Board Web site (http://www.npaihb.org/epi/irb.html) and the IHS Web site (http://www.ihs.gov/MedicalPrograms/Research/irb.cfm).

## TRIBAL COMMUNICATION STRATEGIES

A different worldview affects communication for the researcher within the tribal community. As stated by the authors of the Swinomish Tribal Mental Health Project:

> Indian people are less likely to perceive the world as falling into discrete categories (e.g. physical, social, mental) and more likely to perceive an underlying unity or interaction between all aspects of life. ... Non-Indians tend to separate these aspects of life and treat them as distinct realms having little to do with one another (Clarke 1991, p. 126).

Indians tend to see the world as a continuum—interconnected, as interacting parts of a whole compared with the Western linear viewpoint. Because many misunderstandings arise from this difference in perspective, it is important for the researcher to learn some basic communication strategies.

AIAN populations are often culturally and linguistically different. Currently, there are over 200 different and distinct languages spoken by tribes in the United States, down from over 400 languages just within the last century (Verano and Ubelaker 1991). Cultures and tribes vary from Plains Indians to coastal Indians to woodland Indians to the desert Indians and farmers of the Southwest. There are matriarchal and patriarchal societies, and there are egalitarian and authoritarian societies. The differences are numerous (Verano and Ubelaker 1991), but there are some basic cultural and societal nuances and mores that translate across all tribes and Indigenous populations.

Simple courtesy is essential to working in any community regardless of race. It is important to watch the body language and facial expressions of the audience in order to avoid misunderstandings. Unfortunately, watching too closely, even staring into another's face, may be construed as intrusive to AIAN persons. There is a fine line between what is and what is not acceptable behavior; at times it is hard to find the necessary balance. Verbal and nonverbal communication within the Indian community is different than it is in non-Indian communities. Subtle differences in language usage, cadence, and speech patterns are important to the communication process, and lack of awareness of these subtleties can result in miscommunication. Nonverbal communication may be even harder to understand. As any young child on the reservation will note, one can tell when Grandmother is upset by the way she will look down and frown or sit and twist her handkerchief in her hands when she does not want to talk about something in front of strangers. Saying that Indians are stoic and silent is not necessarily true; there are simply different communication behaviors among Indians (Dukepoo 1998). Once accepted by the community, a researcher will find out how silent Indians really are when they start teasing, as teasing and joking are frequently used to show acceptance and are a way to teach acceptable behavior. Silence is also an accepted form of communication. Silences often last longer with Indians than with non-Indians and may serve as a form of respect or a way of testing the individual. The community respects honesty, which helps to build a trusting relationship. Given the complexities inherent in communication, if necessary, a researcher should find someone who is a respected and recognized member of the community who can interpret the culture and language.

Symbols are usually tribe-specific. For example, a dream catcher is not necessarily used in the Northwest, nor does a Kokopelli appear in the Northern Plains. As a researcher's message is presented to the tribal community, one should be as visual as possible but also remember that these communities have an oral tradition. Because of this, "talking circles" are very useful, as discussed later on in Chapter 6. If a researcher is familiar enough with the community to have access to people from the community, there will be a wide communication network to tap into, often called the "moccasin telegraph" (if you are Indian, you will know how fast this can work!). The researcher should always ask how to be respectful when implementing the sharing of critical or important information and should listen for directions from interpreters and community members. This may include utilizing Native-owned radio and newspapers, taking part in community meetings, and presenting to different tribal committees and tribal councils. Most importantly, commitment earns respect. Researchers should not make promises they cannot keep and should keep the ones they do make just as in any other community in which they may work.

As with any other community, tribal groups should be met in their own territory (Clarke 1991). Nothing earns respect faster for the researcher than personally going to meet with the community after traveling a long way to get there. When conducting meetings, having food available is often important if the meeting is around mealtime or snacks if not. The public health nurse and the community health representative (CHR)/aide, not just the physicians, should be contacted when the researcher enters the community. Allied health staffs that spend their time out in the community rather than at the clinic know the community better than do those who spend most of their time in the clinic. Most have areas of the reservation assigned to them and know the families in that area very well (personal experience as a CHR, research interviewer, and tribal health board member).

Time is a different concept to AIANs when it comes to certain events. Family events, such as deaths, births, and tribal anniversaries, are likely to take precedence over meetings and other activities and may interfere with a researcher's schedule (Clarke 1991). Often, if the individual who has died is an elder or previous council member, the tribal offices may close for the funeral and meetings will be cancelled or rescheduled. Offices may also close for significant historical events that occurred within the tribe, such as for the Nez Perce and the Bear Paw Battlefield commemorating the final battle of the Nez Perce War of 1877. The same is true with tribal council meetings. It may also be that the agenda of the researcher and that of the tribe are not the same. Emergent items or events come up that may shove a research project to the back burner, and a given research project may not come up until the next tribal council meeting, forcing rescheduling by the researcher. It is important that researchers remember to always keep in mind that they are working with the tribes and that rescheduling or waiting until later in the day are some of the complications that may result from working with tribes.

There is a push to develop Indian leaders throughout the country; their involvement and participation in research efforts will only improve the quality of the research and help ensure its success, since they know the communities and are familiar with the issues and challenges.

Professional organizations such as the Association of American Indian Physicians, the Native Research Network, the American Indian Science & Engineering Society, and the American Indian Policy Center, and training programs such as the Native Researchers Cancer Control Training Program through the National Cancer Institute and the Native American Research and Training Center at the University of Arizona are recruiting and training AIAN researchers. Many more Indian professionals are ready to be trained and available to take over health and healthcare research if given the opportunity. One campaign by the American Indian College Fund states, "Have you ever seen a real Indian?" The purpose of this campaign is to get others to recognize that strong, successful Indian professionals are ready and able to work and help their communities.

## OWNERSHIP, REPORTING, AND MANAGEMENT OF DATA

Tribes are asserting their sovereignty in research as they have done with government in the health arena and education. This is particularly true when it comes to rightful ownership of research data about their communities. Tribes are beginning to request memoranda of agreement (MOA) or memoranda of understanding (MOU) between the tribe and the researcher, university, state, or federal agency. In these MOAs and MOUs, tribes assert their rights to data ownership. Arizona and New Mexico at the state and university level have MOAs with tribes. Nationally, tribal tobacco support centers, funded by the Centers for Disease Control and Prevention (CDC), have similar agreements between the tribes they serve and the CDC. An issue that came up recently in discussion with the American Indian and Alaska Native Health Research Advisory Council (HRAC; http://minorityhealth.hhs.gov/hrac) and researchers is the policy of the National Institutes of Health (NIH) of requiring data- or resource-sharing agreements for all studies. Discussion with both federal agencies and tribal communities regarding ways to deal with this issue can have an impact on how the community views studies. Confidentiality of data is important to tribes and tribal members. They will want to know (1) who collects the data, (2) who has access to the data, (3) where the data will be stored, and (4) who will own the data. This is similar to what IRBs ask. As mentioned earlier, MOAs and MOUs may solve some of these problems. These four confidentiality issues will need to be clearly outlined in the research proposal and addressed for the community and the IRB. Tribes are starting to ask that the researcher not keep copies of the research data or specimens after they have completed their research. This issue will be addressed later in the book as an aspect of the Havasupai lawsuit.

One issue related to data confidentiality is the difference between tribe-specific data and regional data. Each data source has its own problems and advantages. With tribe-specific data, confidentiality may be breached unless there is a means to protect the name of the tribe. Identification of an individual may be possible if the tribe is identified because of the small population numbers of some tribes. Another drawback is that small numbers may not allow for statistical significance. However, tribes differ in ways that affect data interpretation that regional data will not be able to address. While regional data provide the advantage of larger numbers and data aggregation, there are other implications. As tribes take over responsibility for their own healthcare, they may use a different data system than the IHS. If IHS no longer collects data for a tribe and that tribe no longer shares their data with IHS, IHS regional data will be incomplete.

The tribes are required to maintain a minimum data reporting system for "health status and services delivery and may only impose minimal burdens on the self-governance tribes" (Federal Register 2002) and only from existing data sets that the tribes already collect as part of their service delivery. They are not required to report these data to any other government agency including IHS. They may opt to participate in a national uniform data set with IHS, but it is a voluntary process (Federal Register 2002). The national data set would be

> to comply with sections 513 [25USC 458aaa-12} and 514 [25 USC. 458aaa-13] of the Act as well as to assist IHS in advocating for the Indian health system, budget formulation, and other reporting required for statute, development of partnerships with other organizations that benefit the health status of Indian tribes, and sharing of best practices" (Federal Register 2002).

Most large aggregate data sets only look at state-by-state data and not at tribe-specific data. There are few data out there that examine the morbidity aspects of AIAN health; most examine mortality only. Existing data typically do not address the issue of the urban population nor do they fully address the reservation population. Additionally, data that are available may be unreliable owing to misclassification of race on the birth or death certificate, as discussed in Chapter 2. These are just a few of the problems related to tracking AIAN status.

Data provided by IHS are complete for its service user population but do not address the issue of those living off reservation or those who do not use the services but still reside on reservation. The data do have an advantage of being consistent over time, able to monitor trends in the population, and capable of making regional/tribal comparisons instead of always aggregating the data into national trends. This is particularly helpful for tribes that need tribe-specific data. Because IHS is underfunded, more tribes are forced to apply to institutions other than IHS to fund their prevention needs. In so doing, they have discovered the value of tribe-specific data in making their case for needed funding, as patterns of need for one tribal community may be masked when aggregated with tribes who don't experience the same magnitude of a problem. Unfortunately, the small population numbers make most tribe-specific data impractical to analyze and use.

As pointed out by Dixon et al. (2001), more and more tribes will compact and the effect of the policy changes will become more evident. As a result, it is important to examine the effects of these changes and plan ahead to provide the best possible guidelines and practices for tribes as they compact and take over more of their own healthcare with the goal of ensuring healthier communities.

One of the most important aspects of doing research in Indian country is presenting the results back to the tribal council, their representatives (which may be organizations such as NPAIHB or AATCHB), or the tribal community through community meetings, local media, and written reports. The tribes can then use the data to guide program development, policy, and planning. Some tribes are now asking that either tribal members or the tribe be included as co-authors on reports or for recognition of specific persons for their assistance in the research effort. Other tribes do not wish their names to be included on the research efforts and may prefer to be mentioned in a manner that does not identify them (e.g., "a tribe in the southwest"). It is important to respect their wishes in either including or excluding them in the publications.

## IMPLICATIONS OF RESEARCH COLLABORATION

Each collaborator, including the tribe, the researcher, and the funding agency, operates under a unique set of experiences and perceptions. For instance, smaller tribes perceive that larger tribes get more attention, funding, and resources, and that the rewards are often limited to those with connections, not ability. The reality is that resources are limited. Some tribes do get larger shares of funds simply by virtue of population size, but when resources are examined by allocation of funds to population size, the ratio of funds to population are usually proportional (Roberts and Jones 2004, Dixon et al. 2001). Regardless, when tribes are involved in research, their involvement translates to increased benefits, including increased funding opportunities and direct access to current research, which helps develop tribe-specific interventions.

Tribes need to participate fully in strategic areas of decision-making at the national, regional, and local levels to promote their research needs. By building coalitions, networks, and partnerships with government agencies and non-federal organizations (i.e., academic or private foundations), tribes become a part of the agenda-setting process. Tribes need to carefully consider benefits and risks of research and decide accordingly before granting approval. There are inherent risks or benefits in all research, and careful consideration of both is important. The Model Research Code (http://www.ihs.gov/ NonMedicalPrograms/Research/irb.htm) can help a tribal community determine a research agenda through careful selection of the components appropriate to that tribe (American Indian Law Center, Inc. 1999). American Indian Law Center, Inc., wrote the code not to be specific to all tribes but as a manual for the tribes to take what they need and apply it to their own situation. The code can be implemented through either a research program or ordinance and provides a model for tribes to use and modify for their use (Deloria PS, personal communication, IHS Research Conference, 2012).

The researcher's learning curve is reduced, as is research approval time, if he or she is involved with the tribes from the beginning (Kaufert et al. 1999). Tribal involvement will also increase the likelihood of research completion.

This style of researcher enjoys greater access to tribes and can become known as a researcher who is willing to work with tribes. The researcher can also build the capacity of the tribe by including them in all phases of the research process. Investing time and effort in mentoring Native students and local researchers builds tribal capacity and will result in local leaders who can design, implement, and disseminate research within their own communities (Bodeker et al. 2002). Involvement also builds trust and shortens approval time within the community. Some researchers report that it takes as long as two to three years to get tribal approval for their research project, which brings us to the issue of funding agencies.

Funding agencies, whether governmental or nongovernmental organizations, need to understand the realities of research in tribal communities. They must revise their guidelines to create partnerships between tribes and researchers by allowing sufficient time for the tribal approval process for proposals or applications. They also need to consider funding tribes directly rather than funding them through state or other federal agencies as cooperative relationships between tribes and these agencies do not always exist. Funding agencies also need to require researchers to report back to tribes in order to create an atmosphere of trust among the funding agency, the researcher, and the community. In past decades, research results were rarely reported back to the tribal communities. It is only recently that funding agencies began requiring researchers to disseminate their results. Many researchers translate that to mean publishing results in the latest medical or public health journal and not taking the results (as they should) to the community either through understandable reports, radio interviews, public announcements, or recommendations for improvement to the tribal council. Native communities, tribes, and Native researchers are starting to see consideration of these issues as more funding opportunity announcements are released specifically for AIAN persons and Native Hawaiians in order to reduce disparities in these populations.

## SUMMARY

Without background information, researchers and funding agencies do not understand tribes' and tribal peoples' viewpoints. Researchers and funding agencies need to understand the history of distrust of tribes and tribal people toward outside researchers. Lack of trust and historical methods of research that violate the rights of human participants are two of the strongest barriers to research in tribal communities. This distrust derives from a variety of causes, including the "gift" of blankets infected with smallpox to tribes, a memory that is only a few generations old (Patterson and Runge 2002). As discussed in Chapters 1, 6, 7, and 8, medical procedures and research have been conducted without consent, often to the detriment of the tribal community. Evidence of research or medical practices that were not tested or condoned by the larger medical community left a bitter taste in the mouths of most tribes (Lone Dog 1999). For example, the current Human Genome Project raises issues within tribal communities that go far beyond previous research considerations. The pros and cons are debated by Native and non-Native researchers alike, and the debate may go on for years. In 1998, the late Dr. Frank Dukepoo, one of only three AI geneticists at the time of his death, outlined tribal opposition to genetic patenting, creation of cell lines, transgenic experimentation, and cloning, and provided pros and cons to conducting genomic research within tribal communities (Dukepoo 1998). Dukepoo, Lone Dog, and Davis contest the ethics of genetic research as it now stands and suggest that it is unacceptable to conduct such research without specific guidelines (Dukepoo 1998, Lone 1999, Davis 2004). Lone Dog and Davis liken the current application of genetics to the theft of land, culture, and traditional knowledge that accompanied European colonization (Lone 1999, Davis 2004). This paternalistic attitude of ownership by non-Natives does not sit well with Native American people. An example of this paternalistic attitude can be seen in a 2004 editorial in *Nature*, in which the author suggests that the Havasupai of Arizona are chasing away "sensitive, caring scientists" from doing research in AIAN communities and that "given the broader potential benefits of research, this cannot be a climate that tribes wish to foster" (Tribal Culture Versus Genetics 2004). While the author of the article suggests that reaching out to each other is good and bringing in Native researchers would help solve the problem, his or her attitude is inappropriate because from the tribal point of view, it is another example of a paternalistic attitude prevalent among non-Indians of "knowing what is best" for the Native community. These are a few examples of the ways that lack of communication and trust have occurred and still occur. Although some of these examples are historical and recent generations were not always directly affected, tribal memory of the breaches of trust remains and passes from generation to generation (Norton and Manson 1996).

Other Indigenous people around the world including those in Canada, New Zealand, and Australia have developed their own research guidelines, with some doing so as early as the 1970s (Humphrey 2001, Scott and Receveur 1995, Ten 2005, Anderson et al. 2003, Eades and Read 1999, Gillam and Pyett 2003, Grove et al. 2003, Sporle and Koea 2004, and Fluehr-Lobban 2000). These strategies and efforts to include Indigenous populations in the development of research have reached across disciplines into areas other than health, including anthropology (Reading 2003). Unfortunately, as Humphrey points out, what started out for Australia as a set of rules and standards quickly devolved to guidelines and became even further "watered down" into priorities (2001). Limitations to these guidelines are becoming apparent as the initial commitment to inclusive and participatory research fades or changes. A broad spectrum of opinions has developed over the years about what needs to be done with these guidelines and how they need to be enforced, or whether they even need to be enforced (Fluehr-Lobban 2000). Humphery (2001) points out the need for a shift not only in the local and researcher awareness of research in Indigenous populations but also for an institutional shift so agencies may affect policy at their level. While the commitment has changed over the years, we can learn from Canada, a country that solidified its commitment to Indigenous research with the development of the Canadian Institutes of Health Research Institute of Aboriginal Peoples' Health. This institute has established two MOUs, one with Australia and New Zealand and another with the United States, to cooperate on Indigenous health research (Cunningham et al. 2003, Sporle and Koea 2004). These agreements serve as an example of "the best of all possible worlds" with the acknowledgment and involvement of the Indigenous population in the research agenda.

The good news is that there is an increased attention to minority/ethnic research and the disparities that exist between these populations and that of the majority group. Federal agencies are increasing their efforts to consult with tribes and tribal organizations. President Clinton issued a memorandum in 1994 requiring departments within the government to consult with tribes on issues that affect them. This policy has been updated several times and can be accessed at http://www.hhs.gov/iga/tribal/report.html. The Office of Minority Health held a conference on health disparities in American Indian and Alaska

Native Health (Denver, CO; September 22–26, 2002), which examined the research issues and in which each region held consultation with the tribes in their respective area. Each of these efforts shows a commitment to the efforts to reaffirm the steps taken previously by President Clinton to reestablish and maintain the consultation with tribes. President Obama (2009) reaffirmed his commitment to President Clinton's original memorandum and states:

> History has shown that failure to include the voices of tribal officials in formulating policy affecting their communities has all too often led to undesirable and, at times, devastating and tragic results. By contrast, meaningful dialogue between Federal officials and tribal officials has greatly improved Federal policy toward Indian tribes. Consultation is a critical ingredient of a sound and productive Federal-tribal relationship.
>
> My Administration is committed to regular and meaningful consultation and collaboration with tribal officials in policy decisions that have tribal implications including, as an initial step, through complete and consistent implementation of Executive Order 13175. Accordingly, I hereby direct each agency head to submit to the Director of the Office of Management and Budget (OMB), within 90 days after the date of this memorandum, a detailed plan of actions the agency will take to implement the policies and directives of Executive Order 13175. This plan shall be developed after consultation by the agency with Indian tribes and tribal officials as defined in Executive Order 13175. I also direct each agency head to submit to the Director of the OMB, within 270 days after the date of this memorandum, and annually thereafter, a progress report on the status of each action included in its plan together with any proposed updates to its plan.

As each agency submits their plans for these consultation efforts, it provides tribes an opportunity to address some of the issues needed in Indian country. The tribes also have an opportunity to provide input into these documents as the government holds consultation sessions at the National Congress of American Indians, the AIAN HRAC, and other forums.

In a speech on January 14, 1879, to President Rutherford B. Hayes, cabinet members, Congress, diplomats, generals and others, Chief Joseph requested that the exiled Ni Mii Pu (Nez Perce Tribe) be allowed to return to their traditional lands. He stated:

Treat all men alike. Give them all the same law. Give them all an even chance to live and grow. All men were made by the same Great Spirit Chief. They are all brothers. The earth is the mother of all people, and all people have equal rights upon it (Chief Joseph 1879).

Chief Joseph's words beautifully express what American Indians and Alaska Natives seek—to be treated equally and to be given the same rights to health and happiness as others have and the legal protection to seek and secure these rights.

## REFERENCES

American Academy of Pediatrics Committee on Native American Child Health; American Academy of Pediatrics Committee on Community Health Services. 2004. Ethical considerations in research with socially identifiable populations. *Pediatrics.* 113:148–51.

American Indian Law Center, Inc. 1999. *Model Research Code.* Albuquerque, New Mexico: American Indian Law Center, Inc. Available at: http://www.ihs.gov/Research/ pdf/mdl-code.pdf. Accessed September 15, 2013.

Anderson I, Griew R, McAullay D. 2003. Ethics guidelines, health research and Indigenous Australians. *N Z Bioeth J.* 4(1):20–9.

Bodeker GG, Kronenberg F. 2002. A public health agenda for traditional, complementary, and alternative medicine. *Am J Public Health.* 92(10):1582–91.

Bruyneel K. 2007. *The Third Space of Sovereignty: The Postcolonial Politics of U.S. Indigenous Relations.* Minneapolis: University of Minnesota Press.

Chief Joseph. 1879. *That All People May Be One People, Send Rain to Wash the Face of the Earth.* Kooskia, ID: Mountain Meadow Press.

Clark DH, Holtzman D, Cobb N. 2003. Surveillance for health behaviors of American Indians and Alaska Natives: findings from the Behavioral Risk Factor Surveillance System, 1997–2000. *MMWR Morb Mortal Wkly Rep.* 52(SS07):1–13.

Clarke JF, editor. 1991. Swinomish Tribal Mental Health Project. *A Gathering of Wisdoms, Tribal Mental Health: A Cultural Perspective.* La Conner, WA: Swinomish Tribal Community.

Cunningham C, Reading J, Eades S. 2003. Health research and Indigenous health. *BMJ.* 327(7412):445–7.

Davis DS. 2004. Genetics: the not-so-new new thing. *Perspect Biol Med.* 47:430–40.

Dixon M, Mather DT, Shelton BL, et al. 2001. Economic and organizational changes in healthcare systems. In: Dixon M, Roubideaux Y, editors. *Promises to Keep: Public Health Policy for American Indians and Alaska Natives in the 21st Century.* Washington DC: American Public Health Association.

Dukepoo FC. 1998a. Genetic services in the new era: Native American perspectives. *Community Gene.* 3:130–3.

Dukepoo FC. 1998b. The trouble with the Human Genome Diversity Project. *Mol Med Today.* 4(6):242–3.

Eades SJ, Read AW. 1999. The Bibbulung Gnarneep Project: practical implementation of guidelines on ethics in Indigenous health research. *Med J Aust.* 170(9):433–6.

Title 42: Public Health (42 CFR) part 137 – Tribal Self-Governance. *Federal Register.* 67:96; May 17, 2002.

Fluehr-Lobban C. 2000. Globalization of research and international standards of ethics in anthropology. *Ann N Y Acad Sci.* 925:37–44.

Fouquera R. 2001. *Urban Indian Health.* The Henry J. Kaiser Family Foundation. Available at: http://www.kff.org/minorityhealth/loader.cfm?url=/commonspot/security/getfile.cfm&PageID=13909. Accessed October 30, 2010.

Gillam L, Pyett P. 2003. A commentary on the NH&MRC draft values and ethics in Aboriginal and Torres Strait Islander health research. *Monash Bioeth Rev.* 22(4):8–19.

Grove N, Brough M, Canuto C, et al. 2003. Aboriginal and Torres Strait Islander health research and the conduct of longitudinal studies: issues for debate. *Aust N Z J Public Health.* 27(6):637–41.

Humphrey K. 2001 Dirty questions: Indigenous health and "Western research." *Aust N Z J Public Health.* 25(3):197–202.

Indian Health Service, Division of Program Statistics. *Regional Differences in Indian Health 2002–2003.* Available at: http://www.ihs.gov/dps/index.cfm?module=hqPubRD03. Accessed September 28, 2013.

Kaufert JM, Kaufert PL. 1998. Ethical issues in community health research: implications for First Nations and circumpolar Indigenous peoples. *Int J Circumpolar Health.* 57(1):33–7.

Kaufert J, Commanda L, Elias B, et al. 1999. Evolving participation of aboriginal communities in health research ethics review: the impact of the Inuvik workshop. *International J Circumpolar Health.* 58:134–44.

Kickingbird K. 2000. The relations of Indian nations to the US government. In: Rhoades ER, editor. *American Indian Health, Innovations in Healthcare, Promotion and Policy.* Baltimore, MD: The Johns Hopkins Press.

Liao Y, Tucker P, Okoros CA, et al. 2004. REACH 2010 Surveillance for health status in minority communities—United States, 2001–2002. *Morb Mortal Wkly Rep.* 53(SS06): 1–36.

Lone Dog L. 1999. Whose genes are they? The Human Genome Diversity Project. *J Health Soc Policy* 10:51–66.

Manson SM, Garroutte E, Goins RT, et al. 2004. Access, relevance, and control in the research process: lessons from Indian country. *J Aging Health.* 16: 58S–77S.

Medicine B. 1996. *Encyclopedia of North American Indians – Women.* CENGAGE Learning. Available at: http://college.hmco.com/history/readerscomp/naind/html/ na_043400_women.htm. Accessed October 30, 2010.

Norton IM, Manson SM. 1996. Research in American Indian and Alaska Native communities: navigating the cultural universe of values and process. *J Consult Clin Psychol.* 64(5):856–60.

Obama B. 2009. *Presidential Memorandum for the Heads of Executive Departments and Agencies: Tribal Consultation.* Available at: http://www.whitehouse.gov/the-press-office/ memorandum-tribal-consultation-signed-president. Accessed October 30, 2010.

Patterson KB, Runge KT. 2002. Smallpox and the Native American. *Am J Med Sci* 323(4):216–22.

Powell JF, Jerome RC. 1999. *Chapter 2, Report on the Osteological Assessment of the "Kennewick Man" Skeleton.* Archeology & Ethnography Program. Available at: http:// www.cr.nps.gov/archeology/kennewick/#non-destr. Accessed October 30, 2010.

Pyett P. 2002. Working together to reduce health inequalities: reflections on a collaborative participatory approach to health research. *Aust N Z J Public Health.* 26: 332–6.

Reading J. 2003. The Canadian Institutes of Health Research, Institute of Aboriginal People's Health: a global model and national network for Aboriginal health research excellence. *Can J Public Health.* 94(3):185–9.

Roberts J, Jones JD. 2004. Health disparities challenge public health among Native Americans. *Northwest Public Health.* 21(2):8–9.

Scott K, Receveur O. 1995. Ethics for working with communities of Indigenous peoples. *Can J Physiol Pharmacol.* 73(6):751–3.

Sebelius K, Roubideaux Y, Church R, Paisano E. 2003. *Trends in Indian Health 2000–2003 Edition.* Available at: http://www.ihs.gov/publicinfo/publications/trends98/front. pdf. Accessed October 30, 2010.

Sharp RR, Foster MW. 2002. An analysis of research guidelines on the collection and use of human biological materials from American Indian and Alaskan Native communities. *Jurimetrics.* 42:165–86.

Smith LT. 2012. *Decolonizing Methodologies: Research and Indigenous Peoples.* 2nd edition. London, UK: Zed Books LTD.

Smith P. April 17, 2012. Testimony to Department of Health and Human Services, National Center for Vital and Health Statistics, Subcommittee on Privacy, Confidentiality, and Security. Available at: http://www.ncvhs.hhs.gov/120417tr.htm. Accessed September 11, 2013.

Sporle A, Koea J. 2004. Maori responsiveness in health and medical research: clarifying the roles of the researcher and the institution (part 2). *N Z Med J.* 117(1199):U998.

Ten Fingers K. 2005. Rejecting, revitalizing, and reclaiming: First Nations work to set the direction of research and policy development. *Can J Public Health.* 96(1):S60–3.

Tokunaga K, Ohashi J, Bannai M, et al. 2001. Genetic link between Asians and Native Americans: evidence from HLA genes and haplotypes. *Hum Immunol.* 62(9):1001–8.

Tribal culture versus genetics [editorial]. *Nature.* Available at: http://www.nature.com/ nature/journal/v430/n6999/full/430489a.html. Accessed July 15, 2013.

US Department of Health and Human Services. 1994. *Working Group Report On Consultation With American Indians And Alaska Natives.* Available at: http://www.ihs. gov/adminmngrresources/regulations/deptpolicy.asp. Accessed July 15, 2013.

US Department of Health and Human Services. 2009. Code of Federal Regulations. Title 45 Public Welfare, and Part 46 Protection of Human Subjects. Available at: http://www. hhs.gov/ohrp/humansubjects/guidance/45cfr46.html Accessed October 30, 2010.

# 4

# The Importance of Cultural Competency: Understanding the Limits of the Outsider's Knowledge

Jennie R. Joe, PhD, MPH

## INTRODUCTION

There appears to be little disagreement about the desirable skills and knowledge to be included in a training program or a curriculum for developing cultural competency, especially for service providers and others who expect to work with diverse, multicultural populations. However defined, most of these desirable skills and knowledge are also part of a national agenda in the healthcare and health research arenas. Many of those teaching these skills are people with previous cross-cultural experience who are helping to meet the United Nations Educational, Scientific and Cultural Organization (UNESCO) 2001 goal to increase the cadre of culturally competent healthcare providers and researchers to respond more effectively to the complexity of health problems confronting the ever-growing diversity of cultures in the United States (UNESCO 2001).

Within this agenda, the need for cultural competency is well articulated. However, there is less agreement about how best to acquire or to assess cultural competency of those trained and the ultimate impact on the health status outcome of those they serve, primarily because there is no standard criterion to delineate what levels of cultural competency skills or knowledge is needed to see its impact.

To date, what is clear is that those considered most appropriate to take these professional development courses are primarily members of the majority culture who are encouraged to learn about various cultural groups and how these groups' health beliefs, health behaviors, or language barriers affect their responses to healthcare services and disease prevention efforts. Cultural competence, therefore, has been added to the tool kit for those engaged in addressing a number of health disparities confronting racial and ethnic communities. The need for cultural competency, however, should be mandatory for all those engaged in community-based activities involving diverse communities. In addition to healthcare providers, cultural competency is also critical for researchers engaged in studies of these groups, particularly community-based participatory research (CBPR), a research agenda that calls for close collaboration and partnership with the cultural groups participating in the research activity.

Enhancing cultural competency of service providers and researchers who are themselves members of minority cultures is encouraged because many recently trained minority scholars and service providers are most likely to have lived outside the experiences of their grandparents or outside the cultural enclaves of their families. As with their non-minority peers, most minority service providers and scholars receive their academic training and professional socialization outside their own racial or ethnic communities. As a result, many are not fluent in the language of their families and face many of the same challenges that are experienced by their peers from the majority culture when they interact with their own ethnic communities.

In this chapter we provide a brief analysis of what cultural competency is and how it can be used to enhance the research experience for the researcher and his or her respective community research partners. Cultural competency in and of itself is an ongoing learning process that ultimately benefits both the researcher and the community in which the research is conducted.

## CULTURAL COMPETENCY DEFINED

Developing, measuring, and defining cultural competence remains problematic. Understandably, no one expects that all those who complete training will be immediately culturally competent. It does mean, however, that the training or awareness provided should aid the trainees not only to reflect on their own culture but also to observe and respect key cultural rules that are important and applicable to their situation. In many cases, cultural awareness may be learned in the classroom, but cultural competency is gained from experience.

The complexity of cultural competence is best illustrated in the following definition used by the Division of Nursing within the Bureau of Health Professions, part of the US Department of Health and Human Services:

> Cultural competence is a set of academic and interpersonal skills that allows the individual to increase their understanding and appreciation of cultural differences and similarities within, among and between groups. This requires a willingness and ability to draw on community-based values, traditions, and customs and to work with knowledgeable persons both of and from community in developing targeted interventions, communications, and other supports (2003).

The preceding definition places emphasis on the individual or the individual's interpersonal skills, but cultural competency is not always limited to the individual; it also can be at the structural level of a healthcare delivery system. Varying levels of cultural competency are viewed as occurring from the broader systems level to the level of the individual (Cross et al. 1989). At the systems level, for example, the attention might be on the institution's efforts to integrate cultural competency training for its staff or improve healthcare access for the underserved by finding ways to break down provider–patient language barriers.

There is no question that the growing complexity of a multicultural society in the United States has emphasized the importance of culture, particularly as it affects health behaviors and health disparities. The importance of culture is given especially high priority in health for a number of racial and ethnic minorities not only because they bear the burden of several health disparities but also because they receive their healthcare from resources that are largely planned, organized, and delivered by members from the majority culture.

The many contributing causes of the prevailing health disparities for several racial and ethnic groups include lack of access to healthcare, distrust of healthcare delivery services, and service providers' lack of cultural knowledge or cultural insensitivity. Examples of the lack of cultural knowledge by service providers includes failure to take into account low health literacy levels that limit knowledge about some of the prevalent health problems, and thereby missing opportunities for needed screening and not recognizing in the diagnostic or treatment plans the possible use of herbal or other Indigenous treatments that might compromise prescribed Western medical treatments (Brach and Fraser 2000).

Encouraging health agencies and staff to develop cultural competency is therefore viewed by multiple entities, including the federal and state governments, as part of the solution to improving health outcomes for patients from different cultural groups. Cultural competency is thus one common thread found among the efforts by the United States to close the gap on several health disparities that are more prevalent among certain racial, ethnic, or underserved groups. There is no question that this shortcoming needs to be addressed and that various strategies such as cultural sensitivity training are desirable and should be encouraged.

## WHAT IS CULTURE?

To understand cultural competency, we must ask the question: what is culture? A term initially coined by anthropologists, "culture" has a range of meanings. For example, two anthropologists, Kroeber and Kluckhohn (1952) reported 164 different definitions of culture, a list that undoubtedly has continued to increase since the 1950s. More recently, the United Nations Educational, Scientific and Cultural Organization (UNESCO) has defined culture as follows:

> Culture comprises the whole complex distinctive spiritual, material, intellectual and emotional features that characterizes a society or social group. It includes not only the arts and letters, but also modes of life, the fundamental rights of the human being, value systems, traditions and beliefs (2001).

The perception of culture as defined by UNESCO is not only comprehensive but also implies that culture is ever changing. Because culture is dynamic, the expectation is that there are both inter- and intra-cultural differences among and within groups, including differences within the same family in which some of the more visible intra-cultural differences may be influenced by intergenerational differences and be the result of the melding of more than one culture as a product of interracial marriage, for example.

Given the complexity of inter- and intra-cultural difference at all levels of society, the goal of achieving cultural competency even within one cultural group can be challenging. Understandably, one can develop competency in certain areas by learning the language of a community, but this accomplishment may not include subtle verbal and nonverbal cues when sensitive information such as personal health beliefs or spiritual practices is being discussed.

## THE FOUR PREREQUISITES FOR CULTURAL COMPETENCY

Papadopouplos and Lees (2002) put forth a model for developing culturally competent researchers which builds on three key concepts developed for teaching service providers cultural competency: cultural awareness, cultural knowledge, and cultural sensitivity. These components are important for researchers and service providers, but cultural competency must also include a fourth element—cultural humility.

### Cultural Awareness

Cultural awareness about a problem in a special population includes knowledge not only about the population but also about the population's ongoing interventions in addressing the problem. For example, if the goal is to develop or examine culturally based substance abuse treatment models, it is important to know about not only the problem of substance abuse and its existing treatment modalities, but also how this problem is defined and treated in the specific community where the study is to take place. The study site's treatment program may be gender or age specific with treatment options that are culturally specific and may include use of local tribal elders or herbalists as well as talking circles in lieu of group therapy. Considerable attention in the research agenda will need to address how best to document or measure treatment outcomes with the use of these culturally specific interventions.

Because the scope of the problems change, as do available resources, collection of qualitative data might be necessary in order to establish the community's current perception of the problem, treatment programs, and other existing interventions or prevention efforts. Framing a community profile also calls for the use of other data such as demographics that help provide age distribution so there is an idea of the risk and mortality linked to the problem to be examined. Qualitative data such as that obtained from focus groups or open-ended interviews can provide useful and valuable data that cannot be obtained from surveys or forced choice answers.

## Cultural Knowledge

Brach and Fraser (2000) rightly note that cultural competence has to go beyond a few courses in cultural awareness or cultural sensitivity. Cultural competency preparation, according to them, should also include learning about values and other factors that influence common health behaviors or practices. If one wants to help change an unhealthy lifestyle, for example, one needs to know both the consequences of risk behavior and how to use cultural knowledge to develop culturally appropriate interventions.

Increased cultural knowledge can also help avoid stereotypes, prejudice, and discrimination. Formal courses or workshops can be helpful, but it is also important to learn from community members. This requires active interactions with community members as well as taking part in various community events. One traditional practitioner (tribal healer) who works extensively with different physicians and other healthcare workers in his community reported recently that his community members feel a strong kinship with one of the non-Native social workers because this service provider participates in community functions and is not afraid to make home visits or follow local custom such as taking meals with the family while on these visits. Because he has made an effort to be a community member, he is not viewed as a social worker, but rather as a part of the community. The practitioner also noted that he and others find this service provider to be approachable, worthy of trust and respect; they are willing to listen to his ideas and recommendations.

Cultural knowledge is an important part of co-learning and can start at the first meeting between a researcher or service provider and the community members. For example, during the first meeting when introductions are made, the researcher should be willing to provide more than just a name and academic credentials. Additional information on personal background, where he or she was born, whether he or she has a family, what work he or she has conducted with other groups in other communities, and other relevant details will help community members feel that they have some context for understanding why the researcher is there and is interested in the community. This kind of disclosure also paves the way for community members to say more about themselves and helps to promote a comfortable interaction.

## Cultural Sensitivity

Cultural sensitivity often refers to being aware of the cultural differences and similarities that exist between the self and others and how these similarities and differences might influence the individual and the group's values and behavior (Cross et al. 1989). Differences such as language or physical appearance are usually apparent during any initial encounter, but other personal characteristics are less visible, such as personal values or beliefs. For example, a researcher's own values and behavior may be especially challenged when the researcher embarks on studies that examine difficult social problems that have the potential to raise sensitive issues for others in the community, such as child abuse, incest, family violence, and intergenerational use of illicit drugs. Without question, many of these social problems exist in a number of communities, and addressing them without sensitivity may result in uncomfortable confrontations that could preclude much needed interventions. Utilizing local partners (including community members) can help identify effective and sensitive ways to address some of these issues. It may also mean enlisting the services of a consultant or two who have participated in or been affected by the problem being examined.

The ultimate goals of culturally competent research efforts are to encourage nonpaternalistic and beneficial working relationships with community partners and to help enhance that community's research capacity, advocacy, and learning. In other words, in these types of research projects, the researcher cannot be detached but needs to actively work with community partners as colleagues to find mutual ways to avoid compromising the research activities as well as to maintain objectivity. Bringing in the different and diverse perspectives of the study population may also include involving racial and ethnic minority researchers, whose perspectives may increase the value of the study findings. Ambramowitz and Murray (1983), for example, found in one experiment that ethnic minority and nonminority researchers who were asked to examine the same research data came up with differing conclusions. Their respective conclusions, according to the authors, were possibly influenced by differences in sensitivity to cultural nuances and differences.

A culturally competent researcher's study must, where appropriate, also address problems related to issues of validity and reliability that can arise when there is little or no preparation for analyzing data collected by bilingual interviewers. Although the analysis process can become more time consuming and complex, Brislin (1993) advises that culturally competent assessment require translations to be checked for equivalency in meaning and measurement and that equivalent meanings be considered, at times, when these do not exist in the tribal language.

An attempt to address validity was an important goal of one Native researcher who recently completed a pilot study on how one type of cancer is perceived by adult tribal members and whether they had been screened or were familiar with various methods of early detection (personal discussions with P. Sanderson, University of Arizona, January 30, 2008). The research design called for use of bilingual data collectors (including the investigator, who was also from the tribe under study) and incorporated a number of data collection methods, including focus groups in selected geographic areas of the reservation. To get to the deeper analysis of the focus group data and to generate consensus on the bicultural themes that emerged, the investigator sought input from three groups of reviewers to examine key themes found in the data: (1) members of the research team, (2) selected community tribal members, and (3) colleagues (Native and non-Native) not involved in the research. While the data analysis on this study is not yet completed, the researcher has commented that this was a useful approach to confirm selected key themes based in part on the language used in expressing cultural perspectives.

This study was not a CBPR project, but was encouraged and supported by tribal leaders because it would provide some relevant information on community members' knowledge and participation in cancer screening. The tribe saw the importance of this study because of the high mortality rate associated with this cancer, which was attributed, in part, to late stage diagnosis and a suspected low level of community awareness on the need for cancer screening. Although there are some regional differences, cancer is one of the leading causes of death for American Indians and Alaska Natives (AIAN; Edwards et al. 2005, Epsey et al. 2007). Cancer and other morbidity and mortality data sources for AIAN persons are not without problems. One of the most common problems encountered is underestimating the prevalence or the mortality associated with various health conditions because of racial misclassification (Indian Health Service 1996). An American Indian at birth may be identified on the birth certificate as an American Indian, but upon death, he or she may be marked as Hispanic or White because of the lack of such a category on the certificate or the prohibition by state laws to record or collect racial and ethnic identification. With this problem in mind, competent researchers engaged in community-based studies (in urban or rural communities) generally have to collect additional data to confirm race, such as language, participation in key traditional tribal ceremonies or activities, and resources utilized in time of illness.

## Cultural Humility

Cultural humility is a process by which one attempts to evaluate his or her own perceptions based on experience in order to expand one's knowledge and improve his or her ability to function more effectively in a different culture (Tervalon and Murray-Garcia 1998). Cultural humility is critical to ensuring effective and respectful ways of addressing or studying critical health concerns that confront different racial and ethnic minority communities. Implicit in this idea is that whether one is from within or from outside the culture of the study group, the researcher needs to be open to learning from these encounters (Weaver 1999). As noted by Hunt (2001), culture does not determine behavior, but rather affords group members a repertoire of ideas and possible actions and also provides them with a framework through which they understand themselves, their environment, and their experiences. Because culture is never static, a researcher needs to understand that what an ethnographer described about a specific cultural community decades earlier may have changed substantially and not be relevant today. Understanding this is important, because some Native peoples view some of these early descriptions as sources of negative stereotypes based on misinformation or misunderstanding by the observer.

It is helpful to know what sources or information the community deems most accurate or acceptable. Today, most tribes have a Web site, local community colleges with ample literature, and possibly local scholars who can provide information. Being open to learning or being a co-learner is a part of developing cultural humility. It forces us to continually challenge our own behaviors, values, perceptions, and experiences. Humility helps us with our ideas and interpretations about others who are "not like us."

A non-Native pediatrician at a recent roundtable discussion said that when she decided to work on the reservation, she asked for and received a list of books to read about the local tribe. She said the books helped her to ask appropriate questions and also helped her get a grasp of the tribal history. She also added that when it comes to patient care, she always tells the patient that she needs his or her help, especially in providing information about the family and the children so that what is decided as treatment will be done in a cooperative environment. She said that this approach towards cultural humility helps her remember that parents are essential players in the care of the child.

Because one cannot be a cultural expert or culturally competent in every situation or with every cultural group, some cultural experts (and in this case, tribal elders and Indigenous researchers) remind young scholars that their journey toward developing cultural competency should begin with humility. In other words, each learns about the other's culture (Tervalon and Murray-Garcia 1998, Freire 1970). Moreover, humility is a value found in many of the teachings of Native cultures, but it is a value that can be easily mistaken for passivity or viewed as a negative attribute, such as when a Native person does not make eye contact or does not immediately engage in conversation. What is perceived as passivity may actually be viewed culturally as a respectful action or taking time to evaluate or "size up" the intent of the interaction. The latter often happens when this initial meeting is with someone such as a physician or researcher who may appear to be in control of the situation. More often than not, however, this "passivity" or quiet reception is a form of respect (Brant 1990).

Cultural humility and cultural sensitivity are dynamic and ever-changing. Tribal heterogeneity serves as a useful reminder that experiences or lessons learned from working with one tribal cultural group may need to be modified when one begins working with another tribal community. Healthcare providers, compared with researchers, are less likely to encounter a greater need to readjust or readapt in a new setting because the services they offer a community or a patient are more easily understood. And because the arrival of researchers or research activities in tribal communities is more recent than that of healthcare providers, researchers do not always fit neatly into the community's experience or are not always acknowledged for possible contribution to improving the health of the community. In fact, as discussed elsewhere in this book, researchers may not be welcomed because of stories heard about former research abuses, even when these abuses may have taken place elsewhere or occurred decades ago when there were no formal policies on the protection of human study participants.

Thus, there is no one Native culture. Although this number will soon increase, there are presently 565 federally recognized AIAN tribes in the United States, each with its own unique culture and language. Tribes may have federal or state recognition. Some of the tribes live in well-defined areas or reservations, while others live in areas that are not easily identified as tribal lands; they reside in communities that are a "checkerboard" of both tribal and non-tribal land. These different environments with diverse populations and resources frequently have an impact on both healthcare services and research strategies. For example, a recruiting or sampling strategy may be a challenge if the reservation community is a patchwork of reservation and private land so that homes of tribal members may not be easily discernable from their non-Indian neighbors. Similarly, AIAN persons residing in cities do not always live in one enclave in an urban area but may instead be scattered from the suburbs to intercity ghettos, depending on the family's financial resources. The urban setting also has the added problem of racial identification, especially since each new generation is likely to be multicultural as well as multiracial as a result of marriage. In most instances, reliance on participants' self-identification is useful but the inclusion of culturally oriented variables in some forms of research may need further examination and clarification.

While institutions that are part of the local healthcare delivery system are usually transparent, some of the challenges in research activities may be less visible. Obviously, the visibility of the healthcare delivery system and endorsement by local governance aids the acceptance of healthcare providers more readily than researchers. The initiation of a study or the presence of a research team may not be readily known or welcomed by the community except by those who have endorsed the study. For example, in some communities, the tribal health committee members or other tribal leaders may be informed and are therefore eager to endorse a study on a topic. But the same initiative may not be supported at the community level because the community sometimes has little or no information as to why the initiative is being proposed. Local opinion leaders who do not hold political office or have an official role may not see the value of studying the prevalence of substance abuse among their youth if there are no services to help the youth. The tribal health leaders, however, may see the value of such a study as a way to document a need for developing services. If a study or program is to be accepted, it must have some visibility by expanding the preliminary discussions (formal and informal) with as many community leaders as possible. Presentations at a community meeting or an article in the local tribal newspaper or announcement on the radio are but a few ways to improve communication about a project or study that is being proposed.

## CULTURAL COMPETENCY ISSUES FOR AMERICAN INDIAN AND ALASKA NATIVE COMMUNITIES

Personnel working for agencies providing education, health, and social services to AIAN persons are generally encouraged to give attention to issues such as language differences, cultural differences, and the need for cultural sensitivity or awareness. Today, these various topics are part of ongoing formal cultural orientation offered at most health facilities, and attendance is required of new employees working with various tribes. Unfortunately, the need for cultural competency in research has yet to become a key concern outside those associated with rules governing the protection of human participants.

Health literacy has and continues to be an important part of the healthcare delivery system for many tribes. Where the need still exists, medical interpreters continue to be a necessity and are essential in helping address problems associated with health literacy or language barriers. In some Native communities, people, especially elders, may only speak their Native language. In addition to trained medical interpreters, another cadre of workers that are essential in the healthcare delivery system in most tribal communities is that of trained paraprofessionals known as Community Health Representatives (CHRs). These individuals serve as a critical liaison between the members of the community and the healthcare delivery system. They are usually tribal members who speak the language and are employed by their respective tribes.

In health-related research projects, skilled CHRs who are bilingual, know the community, are familiar to the families, and have health knowledge are an asset.

Despite the longstanding attention to cultural issues, the need for cultural knowledge and sensitivity is still important as many new service providers as well as researchers (Native and non-Native) brush up against a number of related challenges, including sensitivities derived from sociocultural distinctions as well as the frustrations some AIAN communities feel over the prolonged history of health disparities experienced by their people, especially when previous studies failed to improve the community's poor health circumstances. The tendency to treat tribal communities as convenient research laboratories has also fueled a growing anti-research sentiment in some communities, even when such studies have been perceived or proven to be beneficial to the communities.

It is important to note that the anti-research sentiment does not exist in every tribal community. Some communities are funding their own research, and others have increased their control of research by teaming up with researchers under the umbrella of CBPR. The acceptance of the benefit of research has also increased as the community's control of their health services increases. The growing number of tribal epidemiology centers is but one example of this growing appreciation for public health surveillance and other related health research. Moreover, as tribes take over management of these programs, most make a considerable effort to ensure that the services provided be culturally relevant. Health messages or themes, for example, often incorporate the tribal language as well as familiar cultural icons.

## HEALTH DISPARITIES AND CULTURAL COMPETENCE

Today, healthcare policymakers, providers, and health promotion efforts target selected health disparities for several minority groups in the United States, including AIAN communities. Some of the strategies used in closing the health disparity gaps for certain racial and ethnic minority communities include the honing of cultural knowledge and sensitivity on the part of agencies and service providers to ensure that interventions planned and implemented in multicultural settings will be appropriate and acceptable. How cultural sensitivity and competence are achieved, however, depends on what is taught and what is expected from those who participate in these educational programs (Brach and Fraser 2000).

As mentioned before, some common goals in helping providers reach cultural competency include courses on self-awareness, increasing cultural knowledge, and attention to ethical considerations when working with individuals or groups from various cultural backgrounds (Cross et al. 1989). Some of these courses are taught as part of in-service trainings, and cultural experts deliver others. In examining a compendium of cultural competency initiatives in healthcare undertaken by both public and private organizations, the Kaiser Family Foundation found that both types of organizations were faced with the following common challenges: (1) lack of agreement on the terms, definitions, and core approaches; (2) lack of research on the impact and effectiveness of cultural competency; (3) exclusive focus on people of color rather than the broader diverse population; and (4) lack of funding to implement new initiatives (Rees and Ruiz 2003).

While a number of issues listed above are being addressed by various sources, it is not clear how or to what degree the implementation of cultural competence is making a difference in addressing health disparities. Brach and Fraser (2000) note that most cultural competency techniques and their impact on healthcare service delivery or patient outcomes have not been empirically tested, and they therefore recommend studies that document the efficacy of cultural competency in addressing health disparities.

The cultural competency techniques or approaches reviewed by Brach and Fraser (2000) identify nine activities: (1) use of interpreter services (to improve communication), (2) efforts to recruit and retain minority staff, (3) encouragement of staff training (to increase their cultural awareness, knowledge, and skills), (4) coordination of services with traditional healers (where available and utilized), (5) use of community health workers or trained paraprofessionals (as healthcare liaisons), (6) implementation of culturally competent health promotion initiatives (to encourage risk reduction and promoting healthy behaviors of the targeted population), (7) inclusion of family and community members (when appropriate), (8) increasing immersion into another culture (as a way to increase cultural awareness, etc.), and (9) administrative and organizational efforts at accommodations, which take into account access to care such as facility location, hours of operation, and physical environment.

Some of the above approaches are difficult to achieve, especially in rural isolated communities where many AIAN persons reside. Recruiting and maintaining qualified providers is a challenge as a result of isolation, lack of resources, and low salaries. Geographical barriers and harsh climates hamper or discourage staff retention. For example, in parts of interior Alaska, some villages are only accessible by plane, and most goods, including food, have to be flown in. The transportation cost that is usually added to the price of food can be prohibitive for many families. Lack of adequate housing and public transportation are also barriers. Families with school-age children may find schooling inadequate in most rural isolated communities. Thus, many of the health disparities observed in these regions are affected by other factors over which service providers and researchers have no control, including poverty and limited resources.

## COMMUNITY-BASED PARTCIPATORY RESEARCH: A NEW PARADIGM FOR CONDUCTING RESEARCH WITH TRIBAL COMMUNITIES

As discussed earlier in this book, one serious research abuse experienced by Indigenous communities has been the lack of respect paid to tribal members who contributed to the research effort. These Native colleagues and helpers were rarely acknowledged or given credit as interpreters or key informants in the publications of most of the earlier reports or books (Indian Historian 1973, Macauley et al. 1998; Chino, unpublished manuscript, 1998). Fortunately, this form of research abuse is less frequent now, especially since most tribes now have a say about the research conducted in their communities and the dissemination of the results of these studies. One frequent exception to this has been complaints voiced against a few journalists who published works that did not have the permission or approval of tribal leaders.

The growing acceptance of CBPR by the community, however, is acknowledging the contribution being made by community partners. As noted in this collection, CBPR is an orientation to research that utilizes a number of specific methodological tools in a research activity undertaken with community partners and is grounded in the tradition of action, or applied research, and counters the usual "top-down" study designs (Minkler and Wallerstein 2003). It incorporates the theoretical ideas on co-learning promoted by Freire (1970) and more recently by Smith (1999), who argue for decolonizing the nature of research and challenge Native investigators to become more active in the research process.

Minkler and Wallerstein (2003) define CBPR as a "collaborative approach to research that equitably involves all partners in the research process and recognizes the unique strengths that each brings." In this definition, the term "partners" includes members of the community who bring to the research process community knowledge and cultural competence.

At the center of this growth in the interest and use of CBPR is public and private investment. Increasing numbers of private and public agencies are encouraging CBPR. For example, the National Institutes of Health (NIH) is among those agencies requesting studies utilizing CBPR and requires evidence in the research application of support or partnership with the community. Such indications of support may include a letter of support, a resolution from the tribal government, and in many instances, inclusion of the names of the community partners as co-investigators. In addition, key overseers of research activities at institutions such as the university's institutional review board (IRB) are also asking for evidence that the community involved in the research supports the proposed study.

The number and types of CBPR health-related research activities within Native communities are increasing. One impetus for this increase is attributed to the collaborative arrangement between NIH and the Indian Health Service (IHS) to fund health-related studies under a special initiative—the Native American Research Centers for Health (NARCH). In this arrangement, tribal communities and organizations are the prime recipients of research dollars and are free to subcontract and employ university-based research partners. The following partnership requirement is stated as part of the mission of the IHS Research Program: "....to do and to sustain careful and socially responsible scientific inquiry in the health sciences involving American Indian and Alaska Native people and communities, with maximum tribal involvement in and control over that research" (2008).

Under NARCH, the elements of CBPR call not only for co-investigators from the respective participating communities, but also that research activities involve Native college students, junior investigators, and tribal health or community advisory committees in order to help the communities build their research capabilities. In most cases, the research partnership also encourages the tribe to provide not only input on the specific research agenda, but also on the proposed methodology. When the tribe is the grantee, ownership of the data is decided jointly, as are the responsibilities of joint authorship of publications.

Not every tribal community participates in NARCH studies, but where such activities are taking place, the tribes most engaged are those who have been active in several prior research activities. The academic-based investigators working with these communities also tend to be researchers with ongoing relationships with the community. In addition to giving priority to the types of research that are important to their tribal communities, community leaders also make it known which types of research they want to avoid; these often include genetic studies.

And as noted before, some tribes, even though they did not experience it directly, discourage research because they have heard of examples that involved unethical activities of researchers. In other cases, resistance or distrust of research is based on studies that have projected or reinforced negative stereotypes or have detailed what they consider confidential or sacred information. Other resistance to research participation may be the result of the unequal position a community finds itself in when they participate in studies. The researcher may be viewed by the tribe as having more power than the community members because of the researcher's professional positions and employment with research institutions that may also control the research dollars.

## FORMAL RESEARCH CONTRACT WITH TRIBES

To avoid some of the past mistakes, increasing number of tribes have formalized agreements with academic institutions or research firms through a Memorandum of Understanding (MOU) or a Memorandum of Agreement (MOA). The requirement for an MOU may not be stipulated in every tribe's research policies or protocols but various partnership protocols are usually found in their CBPR partnership agreements with researchers.

Under the umbrella of CBPR, power-sharing issues therefore have been resolved in some cases through MOU between the research institution and the tribal community. The MOU delineates how the work on a study will be shared and clearly identifies the responsibilities of each entity. Some MOU may also include specific steps to aid their community's research capacity calling for inclusion of tribal members as co-investigators, for training a cadre of local interviewers, or for teaching individuals to develop data entry expertise, among other things.

CBPR studies are not ideal in every situation or in addressing every problem. Building trust or developing mutual respect between researchers and the community research partners can be costly and time consuming. Once established, however, a successful partnership is likely to lead to a longstanding positive relationship. Examples of such ongoing community-health research partnerships (albeit not all CBPR) are found in the following tribal communities: (1) the longitudinal study of type 2 diabetes mellitus on the Gila River Indian Community that is in partnership with NIH, specifically the National Institute of Diabetes and Digestive and Kidney Diseases; (2) the longitudinal Strong Heart Study, discussed in Chapter 8 and in Chapter 11, involving a number of tribes in the Southwest, Midlands, and Northern plains; and (3) the Johns Hopkins longstanding presence in the White Mountain Apache community and more recently with other tribes such as the Navajo Nation. Some of these partnerships have ongoing clinical trials and other forms of longitudinal studies.

CBPR study models present some challenges for researchers. For example, academic preparation and professional development of a "good" researcher encourages personal objectivity and other forms of detachment from persons or groups being studied. While detachment is possible in certain types of research, such as large-scale survey studies in which there are no personal contacts, detachment is not possible in CBPR, because the success of a study is often dependent on data collection that requires face-to-face interaction with study participants, and the results of the study are expected to benefit the community that has contributed to the study efforts.

Working in partnership and sharing control over the research process can also be a challenge in CBPR, especially in negotiating data ownership. In academia there is no question about the ownership of research data. The responsibility and ethical use of the data as well as its disposition upon completion of the study are specified by IRBs. The investigators' use of data, especially in publications, is also included as a part of the protocol under academic freedom. The key investigator or investigative team and the investigators' home institution are held responsible for protecting data collected under grants and contracts. In addition, special data sharing with other investigators is also required by federal agencies that award sizable grants to academic institutions.

The control of data is a sensitive topic for Native communities. It is therefore important to have a discussion about data ownership at the planning stage of any proposed study. An open dialogue should focus on what the tribal community expects from the data and how certain data might be used. A part of the data discussion should include how the researcher(s) and the community partners can ensure the protection of confidentiality as required by IRBs and in keeping with the promises of confidentiality made to study participants.

Generally, after a full discussion on use and ownership of data, most community partners usually support steps taken to protect participants' confidentiality and understand why raw data with or without identifiers cannot be made available. Even without identifiers, raw data pose problems when studies take place in communities with small populations, as there is an increased possibility that some participants may be identified. A plan for use of the aggregated data by the community, however, is usually welcome. This data can be used by the community to seek grants or solutions to problems identified by the research. Most community partners also want a copy of the final questionnaire (which they often helped develop), a codebook, and aggregated data or the simple distribution of key results.

Who will be responsible for caring for the data file and how it will be managed is often included in the MOU or contract. In some instances, the community partners may prefer that the investigators from the research institution maintain the data, but when needed, the community could request specific aggregated data. The latter is often the case when the community does not have a "safe" place to maintain or protect such research information. The MOU also usually includes the provision that the investigators will provide a copy of the final report to the community and to study participants who at the time of the interview have requested such a copy. Most CBPR agendas usually include how the results of the study will be disseminated and to whom.

If CBPR is planned and implemented correctly, the community partnership can greatly add to the success of the study outcome. Community partners can provide access to potential study participants and help with the most appropriate process for data collection, assist in framing study questions, and help analyze the data. Because they have the community expertise, community partners can be instrumental in making study designs more meaningful. For example, in a study examining parenting roles and their influences on child development, the community partners may agree that the mother-child dyad is important, but they may also suggest broadening the category of parental responsibilities to include extended kin because this represents a cultural parenting practice that is common in their community.

If the study analysis or interpretation encourages joint partnerships, input from community partners also helps enrich the data because they can expand on an idea expressed by the study participants during a survey or in a focus group that may be missed by a researcher. They might also be able to explain why some participants may view a particular problem or issue in a certain way. For example, a child with a mild learning disability may not be viewed as having a disability because these children are able to function at home, and the disability only becomes an issue when the child is in the school setting. In this example, parents who do not view the condition as a disability when queried may also have different ideas about developmental milestones for their children.

## CULTURAL COMPETENCY AND BIAS IN CONTEMPORARY STUDIES

Many of the barriers in conducting research among Native communities are the result of culturally biased research methodologies. In any research endeavor with Native communities, controlling for bias is therefore critical. Bias can occur at various stages of research, including sampling bias, respondent bias, interviewer bias, and instrumentation bias. Of these various biases, instrumentation bias has probably received the most attention in studies conducted with AIAN populations and represents an area in which cultural competency is essential. For example, in a number of cross-cultural studies that included AIAN persons, results have been questionable because the data relied on results utilizing instruments developed and tested for reliability and validity on the majority culture (Frank-Stromberg and Olsen 2004). Potential cultural bias has to be addressed by researchers when such instruments are to be included in cross-cultural settings. One way to address this problem of bias is to seek input from researchers who are familiar with the minority group's behavior, language, and customs.

Asking the right questions is also necessary. For example, a number of instruments used to measure drinking patterns among members of Native communities do not always take into account cultural issues. A researcher who may have considerable expertise in research on alcoholism but has not had any experience or knowledge of drinking patterns of Native groups may unknowingly collect biased data (Spiegler et al. 1993). For example, Westermeyer (1993) notes that surveys on drinking behavior that ask the respondent only for the number of drinks they consume per day or month may underestimate the extent of binge drinking, a significant form of alcohol abuse found in many Native communities. Conversely, he also cautions that recording only the number of drinks per drinking episode may overlook the extent of chronic daily drinking.

Another common bias in alcohol-related research with Native communities is that researchers often use male norms for examining alcohol-related problems for women when examining patterns of drinking, assuming that drinking behavior and patterns of alcohol abuse for Native women are similar to that of Native males (Wilke 1994). As a result, studies that examine alcohol use patterns among women can be biased, and the data can be interpreted as abnormal. It is important then that researchers need to be sure no bias is threatening their research design as well as the validity of their measurements. Instruments can also miss critical information from not knowing the population. For example, asking individuals about the number of fruits and vegetables consumed may be useful. However, for the impoverished, asking if they have had a meal is far more critical. The same issue applies to homelessness, particularly as it applies to Native communities, where patterns of homelessness differ. In both urban and reservation populations people may sleep on a relative's sofa or floor because that's the only place they have, and they may switch from one friend or relative to another depending on who will take them in. Surveys must be tailored to the community and its values, beliefs, and practices.

Social desirability bias is also a potential problem when respondents want to please the researchers by providing answers the respondents think the researchers want to hear. This effort to please the interviewer is likely to produce data that may mask important information or that can provide a false correlation between key variables. The use of pretests and pilot studies in which instruments are tested with a comparable sample of respondents can help overcome or avoid this problem.

## THE NEED FOR CULTURAL COMPETENCE IN RESEARCH

Papadopoulos and Lees describe a culturally competent researcher as one who is "...able to apply the related skills and knowledge in project design, data collection, analysis, report writing, and dissemination" (2002, p.258). As previously noted, the authors discuss such related skills and knowledge as cultural awareness, cultural knowledge, and cultural sensitivity. Papadopoulos and Lees (2002) also suggest that there are two layers of cultural competence: one that is culture-generic and applicable across different racial/ethnic groups and another that is more culture-specific or applicable to a specific group. It is, however, possible to be culturally competent in a generic way in a number of cross-cultural settings, but a researcher also needs to possess culture-specific competence in order to delineate visible as well as subtle differences pertinent to a particular culture. For example, a Native scholar who has worked in East Los Angeles with a diverse population can be sensitive to the various cross-cultural differences and utilize these differences or similarities in comparing certain data points with his or her own culture.

It has also been proposed by a number of researchers, including Geiger (2001) that not only is cultural competence needed in the research arena but also that such an orientation helps decrease research bias. Porter and Villarruel (1993) also call for appropriate training for researchers in issues related to culture and ethnicity as a way to overcome the unicultural or homogenized perspective in research. Without cultural awareness, researchers will continue to impose their own beliefs, values, and patterns of behavior on other cultures (Leininger 1995).

Realizing cultural competence in research is often difficult, especially when it involves an interdisciplinary research team, as each member of the interdisciplinary team brings into the research setting his or her own personal cultural experiences and varying professional opinions about a proposed study. This added dimension can provide a cross-fertilization of ideas that ultimately strengthens the study. But there may be times when cultural sensitivity is not seen as an important part of the research goals by some members of the study team members, who may object or want to abrogate the community partnership, because they view it as a factor contributing to bias. These kinds of issues will need to be addressed and resolved with the study team as well as with community partners so that collaboration with the partnership can be based on trust and full disclosure from the onset.

## SUMMARY

The journey to become more culturally competent is an ongoing and dynamic process. Most of the points covered in this chapter and the suggestions offered on this topic are not meant to be comprehensive. Conducting research in any community is always challenging because each study or project presents its own unique set of lessons to be learned. All researchers, even those from the within the culture group, need to be mindful of cultural competence and its importance in all community-based studies.

## REFERENCES

Ambramowitz SI, Murray J. 1983. Race effects in psychotherapy. In: Murray J, Abramson PR, editors. *Bias in Psychotherapy*. New York, NY: Praeger; pp. 215–255.

American Institutes for Research. 2002. *Teaching Cultural Competence in Health Care: A Review of Current Concepts, Policies and Practices*. Washington, DC: American Institutes for Research. Available at: http://www.innovations.ahrq.gov/content.aspx?id= 943. Accessed November 12, 2012.

Brach C, Fraser I. 2000. Can cultural competency reduce racial and ethnic health disparities? A review and conceptual model. *Med Care Res Review*. 57(suppl):181–217.

Brant CC. 1990. Native ethics and rules of behavior. *Can J Psychiatry*. 35:534–539.

Brislin RW. 1993. *Understanding Culture's Influence on Behavior*. New York, NY: Harcourt College Publications.

Cross T, Bazron B, Dennis K, et al. 1989. *Toward a Culturally Competent System of Care, Vol 1*. Washington, DC: Georgetown University.

Edwards BK, Brown B, Windo PA, et al. 2005. Annual report to the nation on the status of cancer, 1975–2002. *JNCI*. 97(19):1407–1427.

Espey DK, Wu XC, Swan J, et al. 2007. Annual report to the nation on the status of cancer, 1975–2004, featuring cancer in American Indians and Alaska Natives. *Cancer.* 110(10):2119–2152.

Frank-Stromborg M, Olsen SJ. 2004. *Instruments for Clinical Healthcare Research.* 3rd Edition. Boston, MA: Jones and Bartlett Publishers.

Freire P. 1970. *Pedagogy of the Oppressed.* New York, NY: Continuum International.

Geiger HJ. 2001. Racial stereotyping and medicine: the need for cultural competence. *CMAJ (Ottawa).* 164:1699–1700.

Hunt L. 2001. Beyond cultural competence: applying humility to clinical setting. *The Park Ridge Center Bulletin.*

Indian Health Service. 1996. *Final Report: Methodology for Adjusting IHS Mortality Data for Inconsistent Classification of Race-Ethnicity of American Indians and Alaska Native between State Death Certificates and IHS Patient Registration Records.* Silver Spring, MD: Indian Health Service, Division of Program Statistics.

Indian Health Services Research Program. 2008. Available at: http://www.ihs.gov/MedicalPrograms/Research. Accessed February 4, 2008.

Indian Historian. 1973. *Anthropology and the American Indians: A Symposium.* San Francisco, CA: The Indian Historian Press.

Kroeber AL, Kluckhohn C. 1952. *Culture: A Critical Review of Concepts and Definition.* Cambridge, MA: Peabody Museum.

Leininger MM. 1995. *Transcultural Nursing: Concepts, Theories, Research, and Practices.* New York, NY: National League of Nursing Press.

Macauley M, Commanda LE, Freeman WL, et al. 1998. *Responsible Research with Communities: Participatory Research in Primary Care. NAPCTG Policy Statement.* Available at: http://www.naperg.org/responsibleresearch.pdf. Accessed September 10, 2008.

Minkler M, Wallerstein N. 2003. *Community-Based Participatory Research for Health.* San Francisco, CA: Jossey-Bass; p. 6.

Papadopoulos I, Lees S. 2002. Developing culturally competent researchers. *J Adv Nurs.* 37(3):258–264.

Porter C, Villarruel A. 1993. Nursing research with African-American and Hispanic people: guidelines for action. *Nurs Outlook*. 41:59–67.

Rees C, Ruiz S. 2003. *Compendium of Cultural Competence Initiative in Healthcare*. Menlo Park, CA: The Henry J. Kaiser Foundation..

Smith LT. 1999. *Decolonizing Methodologies: Research and Indigenous Peoples*. London, UK: Zed Books, Ltd.

Spiegler D, Tate D, Aitken S, et al., editors. 1993. *Alcohol Use among U.S. Ethnic Minority Groups*. Research Monograph 18. Rockville, MD: US Department of Health and Human Services.

Tervalon M, Murray-Garcia J. 1998. Cultural humility versus cultural competence: a critical distinction in defining physician training outcomes in multicultural education. *J Health Care Poor Underserved*. 9(2):117–125.

United Nations Educational, Scientific and Cultural Organization (UNESCO). 2001. *Universal Declaration on Cultural Diversity. Adopted by the 31st Session of the General Conference*. Paris, France: UNESCO.

US Department of Health and Human Services. Health Resources and Service Administration. Bureau of Health Professions. 2003. Available at: http://www.bphr.hrsa. gov/diversity/cultcomp.htm. Accessed September 15, 2013.

Weaver HN. 1999. Indigenous people and the social work profession: defining culturally competent services. *Soc Work*. 44(3):217–225.

Westermeyer J. 1993. Methodological issues in alcohol research in ethnic minorities: source of bias. In: Spiegler D, Tate D, Aitken S, et al, editors. *Alcohol Use among U.S. Ethnic Minority Groups*. Research Monograph 18. Silver Spring, MD: US Department of Health and Human Services; p. 461–463.

Wilke D. 1994. Women and alcoholism: how a male-as-norm bias affects research, assessment, and treatment. *Soc Work*. 19:145–149.

# 5

# Understanding Diversity Among Indigenous People: Conducting Research With Native Hawaiians and Pacific Islanders

Maile Taualii, PhD, MPH, Joey Quenga, BA, and Raynald Samoa, MD

## INTRODUCTION

Indigenous people worldwide suffer similar challenges relative to research: (1) a lack of visibility because of issues in data collection, analysis, and reporting; (2) distrust of or disinterest by the community; (3) significant health disparities compared with other racial/ethnic groups; (4) communities with low socioeconomic status; and (5) a history of abuse caused by research. However, there are also distinct issues relevant to Native Hawaiians and Pacific Islanders that include culture, geography, and political and historical differences. Because of this, researchers need to demonstrate cultural competence and build relationships with each specific community group of interest.

Indigenous Pacific people, Native Hawaiians, Chamoru, and American Samoans face a heightened vulnerability as a result of a lack of understanding and awareness by the health and science community of the following issues:

tokenistic inclusion, aggregation with other groups, and decentralization of communities. These issues, combined with all the similar challenges other Indigenous people face, increase the propensity for harm when conducting research for and with Indigenous Pacific people.

This chapter provides researchers with a brief background on Indigenous Pacific people and outlines a few considerations that may be helpful when designing a research study that both contributes to scientific knowledge and is beneficial to the community in which the research is conducted.

## INDIGENOUS PEOPLE OF THE PACIFIC

Collectively, the original peoples of Hawai'i, Guam, and American Samoa can be referred to as US Indigenous peoples of the Pacific and self-identify as Kanaka Maoli, Chamoru, and Samoan, respectively. Collectively, they are classified as Native Americans under the Native American Programs Act of 1974; however, many individual Indigenous Pacific people may not classify themselves as Native Americans.

The estimated total population for Native Hawaiian and Other Pacific Islanders (NHOPI) in their respective homelands and in the United States is in excess of 9 million people. Of this, the 2010 US Census identified 1,274,507 as NHOPI persons living in the United States (Table 5.1). While there may be some discrepancies in the reporting of census data (e.g., Samoan, Micronesian, and Melanesian data classifications), of the numbers presented over 859,000 are Indigenous peoples of the United States, while the remaining 415,192 are US immigrants.

In recognition of the special and unique relationships that all of these Indigenous populations have with the federal government, the secretary of the Department of Health and Human Services (DHHS) has identified all of these groups as having "standing" for consultation within the DHHS. Consultation is a unique government-to-government relationship that exists between the federal government and tribes, grounded in the US Constitution. Numerous treaties, statutes, federal case law, regulations and executive orders that establish and define a trust relationship with Indian tribes and other Native Americans (DHHS 2005).

Table 5.1. US Population Count for Native Hawaiians and Other Pacific Islanders by Indigenous Versus Immigrant Status

| Group | Population |
|---|---|
| **Indigenous** | |
| Chamoru – Indigenous People of Guam | 147,798 |
| Kanaka Maoli – Native Hawaiians | 527,077 |
| Samoans | 184,440 |
| Total Indigenous Pacific Islanders | 859,315 |
| **Immigrant** | |
| Fijian | 32,304 |
| Tahitian | 5,062 |
| Tongans | 57,183 |
| Other Micronesians | 69,535 |
| Other Melanesian | 851 |
| Other Polynesian | 10,078 |
| Other Pacific Islander | 240,179 |
| Total Pacific Islander Immigrants | 415,192 |
| All Pacific Islanders | 1,274,507 |

*Source:* US Census 2010.
**Note:** Numbers include both Census racial categories for NHOPI, alone or combined with another race.

## HISTORICAL RELATIONSHIPS BETWEEN PACIFIC ISLANDERS AND THE UNITED STATES

Samoans from the islands of Tutuila, Manu'a, Rose Atoll, and Swain were brought into the US fabric between 1900 and 1905. The United States occupied these islands as a result of the Treaty of Berlin signed with Germany in 1899. Germany retained control of the Samoan Islands of Savai'i and Upolu, known as German Samoa, until 1918, the end of World War I. At the conclusion of the war, the New Zealand government received these islands and retained control of them until 1962, when it turned them over to a newly created Samoan nation (Spoehr 2006). Today Samoa, consisting of Sava'i and Upolu, is an independent nation while the islands of Tutuila, Manu'a, Rose, and Swain remain the territory of American Samoa. The residents of these islands are US nationals, not citizens, but are considered Indigenous peoples within the US population and are part of the "Native American Pacific Islander" definition (Spoehr 2006).

The Indigenous peoples of Guam and the Mariana Islands, the Chamoru, live on numerous islands scattered across the Western Pacific. At the conclusion of World War II, this entire area either came under the control of the United States as part of a United Nations (UN) trusteeship or as a result of conquest. Guam was taken back into the American sphere from the Japanese in 1944. The relationship between the United States and the other Micronesian Islands under the UN, trusteeship changed as different political states and nations emerged, including the Commonwealth of the Northern Mariana Islands in 1978, the Republic of the Marshall Islands in 1979, the Federated States of Micronesia in 1979, and the Republic of Belau in 1981. With the exception of Guam, which today is a US territory, and the Northern Mariana Islands, which are part of a US Commonwealth, the others are all associated states of the United States. An "associated state" is a partner in a formal, free relationship between a political territory with a degree of statehood and another nation. All such states either are independent or have the potential right to independence. Thus, while Chamoru living in these states today have special standing as a result of the Compact of Free Association, which defines the relationship between the United States and the Federated States of Micronesia, the Republic of the Marshall Islands, and the Republic of Belau, the term *Native American Pacific Islander* is applicable only to those Chamoru from Guam and the Commonwealth of the Northern Mariana Islands (Spoehr 2006).

Native Hawaiians became US nationals in 1898 when Hawai'i was annexed by the United States. While it is unclear how Alaska Natives, American Samoans, and Chamoru felt about becoming American when their respective lands became part of the United States, it is clear that the vast majority of Native Hawaiians had no desire to become part of the country. Petitions were sent to the US Senate signed by more than 98% of the then Native Hawaiian population against annexation (Minton and Silva 1998). Despite this protest, annexation occurred and Hawai'i became a US territory in 1900. Most of Hawai'i's residents, including Native Hawaiians, did not become full US citizens until 1958, when Hawai'i became a state. Today, Native Hawaiians are defined in federal law as "any of whose ancestors were natives of the area which consists of the Hawaiian Islands prior to 1778" (US Code 2011), and they are the largest NHOPI subpopulation, with representation found in all 50 states.

In 1974, in recognition of a unique political status, the US Congress passed the Native American Programs Act of 1974, which for the first time defined American Indians, Alaska Natives, and Native Hawaiians as Native Americans on the basis of being Indigenous peoples of states in the United States. While other federal laws had been previously passed identifying Native Hawaiians as having special status, this marked the first time all three peoples were identified as being Native Americans. This term continues today to be an identifier joining all three populations, although it is neither universally accepted nor used by the three populations themselves. To further add to the confusion, often health researchers publishing their reports use this term to apply only to American Indian and Alaska Native populations. However, at the other end of the spectrum, a number of universities with Native American programs include in those programs Native Hawaiians. In short, there is not a consistent or universally understood definition of the term *Native American*.

The Native American Programs Act of 1974 has been amended to include recognition of the fact that other Pacific Island peoples have a special relationship with the United States. The term *Native American Pacific Islander* has been implemented and is defined, per the act, as "an individual who is Indigenous to a United States territory or possession located in the Pacific Ocean, and includes such individuals while residing in the United States" (p. 18).

## DIMINISHED HEALTH STATUS REPORTING CAPACITY

A description of the current health status of the Indigenous peoples of the Pacific is presently an incomplete narrative. Obstacles in obtaining a full description of these people's current health status include historical convention as well as constraints of research methodology.

### Aggregated Health Statistics for Pacific Islanders and Asian Americans

Historically, the health statistics of US Pacific Islanders have been aggregated with Asian Americans because of the small numbers of Pacific Islanders. Although some believe there is political gain from this practice, there are stark limitations in aggregating data in order to describe the health status of US

Pacific Islanders. The common practice of aggregating data—bundling of statistics for projects—has come under fire. This practice displays an inaccurate and misleading picture, which fails to identify particularly vulnerable groups (Taualii 2007). Despite a federal mandate to disaggregate data for Pacific Islanders and Asians, very few national databases that publicly report disaggregated data for the two populations.

### Obesity and Diabetes Prevalence Rates Using Disaggregated Data

Smaller statewide surveys have reported disaggregated information in California and Hawai'i. According to the *State of Asian American, Native Hawaiian and Pacific Islander Health in California Report*, the rate of overweight and obesity in the general population was 56%. Asians were found to have the lowest rates, while the highest rate of all racial/ethnic groups of 70% were found in NHOPI persons (Ponce et al. 2009). Similar results were reported from Hawai'i as well (Hirokawa et al. 2004).

Recent studies, described as follows, have shown that the differences in the rates of obesity between Asians and Pacific Islanders may be more than just a genetically determined morphological divergence, but may signify a distinction in the metabolic capacity of these populations inherent to their relative metabolic phenotype. To better understand these distinctions, it is beneficial to distinguish two components of metabolic phenotype. The first is made up of metabolic capacity, referring to the ability of the body to use energy, and derived from the quality of regulatory organs such as the heart, liver, kidney, and pancreas, to maintain homeostasis. The second component of metabolic phenotype is made up of metabolic load, which refers to the homeostatic burden imposed on metabolic capacity (i.e., high carb diet, sedentary lifestyle, and increased fat mass; Ghosh 2003). A study from New Zealand compared the body fat compositions of a group of Asian Indians, Caucasians, and Pacific Islanders based on their relative body mass indices (BMI, defined as weight in kilograms divided by height in meters squared [$kg/m^2$]). The mean BMI for the Asian Indian cohort was 24 $kg/m^2$, the mean BMI for the Caucasian cohort was 30 $kg/m^2$, and the mean BMI for the Pacific Islander cohort was 34 $kg/m^2$ (Rush et al. 2009). These findings propose that there is a difference in the propensity for the different racial groups to accumulate fat stores, which would suggest to some that each group adjusts to a specific metabolic load uniquely based on their relative metabolic capacity. As Pacific Islanders and Asians lie on opposite ends of the metabolic capacity continuum, epidemiology efforts that lump the two groups together will describe an essentially distorted and inaccurate representation of the state of obesity and metabolic disease (such as type 2 diabetes mellitus) of both populations.

Alarmingly high rates of obesity and related disorders have also been reported in US Pacific jurisdictions. In 2004, 47.6% of adults between the ages of 25 and 65 years in American Samoa were reported to have type II diabetes

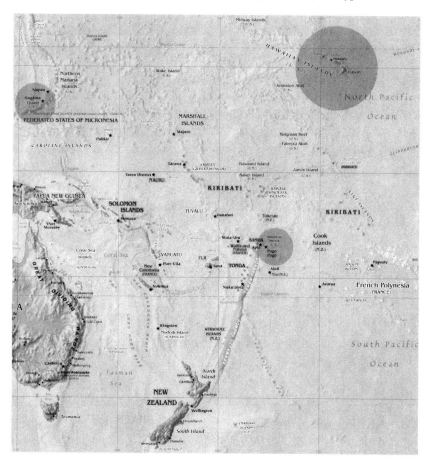

Figure 5.1. Map of the Pacific Ocean. The three circles show where the Indigenous homelands are located for Kanaka Maoli (Hawai'i), Chamoru (Guam) and Samoans (American Samoa).
Source: Google Earth. Pacific Ocean. 2010. Available at: http://www.google.com/earth. Accessed November 12, 2010.

mellitus (Keighley et al. 2007). Studies report temporal trends of increasing diabetes rates of Samoans residing in Hawai'i, Samoa, and American Samoa from the 1970s to 2003. Findings suggest that increasing modernization had a significant influence on the rising rates of obesity and type II diabetes mellitus in Samoans residing in the South Pacific. Except for Hawaiians living in Hawai'i, there is no reported diabetes prevalence for Pacific Islanders residing in the continental United States.

### Limitations of Current Methodologies of Data Collection

The full gravity of the diabetes disparity experienced by the Indigenous Pacific people residing in the United States has not been fully studied owing to several limitations of current data collection methodologies, including limited available data and no existing disease surveillance for the population. The small sample sizes of Indigenous Pacific populations within national data sets do not meet the minimal thresholds for findings to be released. Local and state data may be available in certain areas, but national reports often do not include findings from the Indigenous Pacific population.

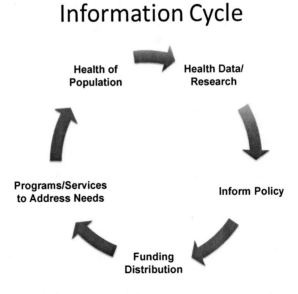

Figure 5.2. Information cycle relationship between data and services.

These current limitations of data collection and epidemiological surveillance directly hinder the efforts of the Indigenous peoples of the Pacific to improve health status, creating a break in the information cycle (Figure 5.2). Limited population data is equivalent with the inability to advocate, thus limiting political power to intervene and garner resources for research grants and programs, which in turn stifles the ability to improve the situation. Although racial differences in health status may seem obvious, the common practice of statistical blending in health studies and the inability to report significant data tends to wash out critical differences that would give public health experts information to develop effective community programs and meaningful research agendas. As mentioned previously, while the disaggregation of Asian and NHOPI data is a federal mandate, it is not enforced or upheld by many federal or local government agencies (Office of Management and Budget 1997; Hoyert and Kung 1997). This refusal to adhere to the federal reporting requirements has had a crippling effect on the NHOPI community, preventing the recognition of population disparities and preventing NHOPI communities from advocating on their own behalf.

## RESEARCH CHALLENGES

Like many Native communities, Indigenous Pacific people face a number of challenges related to research. The challenges that face all small communities resonate with Indigenous Pacific people, for example, being overburdened or over-researched, not having enough resources to support community needs, being unable to direct the research process, and having low numbers of Native scientists. In addition to common challenges, there are a number of additional challenges that are specific to Indigenous Pacific people. The following sections describe these challenges.

### Data Aggregation within NHOPI Category

In addition to the previously mentioned issue of aggregation of NHOPI data with Asians, Indigenous Pacific people face an additional data aggregation challenge. The NHOPI race category definition combines Indigenous peoples of the United States with Pacific Islander immigrants to the United States. Political relationships, health determinants, and access to health services are just a few examples of differences that divide these people.

## Geography

Even on island homelands, Indigenous people are often only a fraction of the total island population. Native Hawaiians constitute only 19.8% of the total population of Hawai'i and the Chamoru constitute 40% of the population of Guam. In American Samoa, however, Samoans are the majority group, at 95% of the total population. For various reasons, a substantial percentage of the population choose to leave their traditional homelands; 43% of Native Hawaiians are on the continent, 43% of Chamoru no longer reside in Guam or in the Northern Marianas, and 72% of Samoans no longer live in American Samoa (US Census 2010). As these groups relocate from their island homes, they experience substantial changes in lifestyle because of limited or reduced access to traditional food, culture, and extended families. However, Indigenous Pacific people often relocate to areas where there are established Pacific Islander communities, which helps to at least partially recreate the island home environment. The top five states to which Indigenous Pacific people relocate are Hawai'i (for American Samoans and Chamoru), California, Washington, New York, and Florida (US Census 2010). While there are states in which there are a greater percentage of Indigenous Pacific people and relationships are developed and the people gather together for events, there are no known Indigenous Pacific neighborhoods. This must be taken into consideration when attempting to recruit Indigenous Pacific people into studies in these locales.

Most surveillance methodologies rely on random sampling to ensure the applicability of the data collected to the general population of interest. To avoid the possibility of selection bias, potential participants are identified via a centralized health care system by singling out common surnames of the community being studied. Although these approaches have been very effective in collecting data in the general population, there are major restraints in implementing them with Indigenous Pacific people. First, no predominant central health care system has been identified for Indigenous Pacific people. Second, the large percentage of Indigenous Pacific people that do not partake in routine health maintenance for economic or personal reasons makes it difficult to accurately describe the health of this community. Likewise, using local phone directories to search for surnames is a complicated procedure. The occupation of a number of Pacific islands by the United States, Germany, Spain, and the United Kingdom as well as frequent interracial marriage of

Natives with immigrants from Asia have made European, Spanish, and Asian surnames common in the Pacific. Thus, identifying only traditional surnames will exclude a large percentage of the population.

The most effective way to recruit Indigenous Pacific people into research studies for non-Indigenous Pacific people is to partner with Pacific Islander organizations, churches, or cultural groups. Partnership with such groups can also support a community-based participatory research (CBPR) process in which Indigenous Pacific people help guide, develop, and control research efforts.

### Federal Travel Limitation

Another major challenge faced by Indigenous Pacific people is also geographic. Pacific island homes are beautiful and sought after by many looking for a tropical vacation. In Hawai'i alone there were approximately 7.2 million visitors in 2011 (Hawai'i Tourism Authority 2011). Because of its beauty and status as a tourist destination, there is an inaccurate belief that official business can not be conducted effectively in the islands. In 2006 and 2008, directives were put in place during the Bush Administration limiting travel to select destinations by government agencies and federal officials (Berkley and Titus 2009). These directives prohibit or limit Hawai'i's ability to host federally sponsored conferences, coordinate site visits from federal project officers, and compete for hosting meetings and conferences.

### Tokenism

Along with the grouping of Pacific Islanders into the category with Asians, another common grouping is combining American Indians, Alaska Natives, and Native Hawaiians. This grouping can be seen in research organizations, caucuses, or service agencies. While this grouping may be well intentioned and supportive of efforts to advocate for Indigenous people in the United States, it can also be a challenge to Indigenous Pacific people. In some cases, the inclusion of Native Hawaiians or other Indigenous Pacific people are listed in the by-laws and mission statements of organizations; however, there may be no genuine effort to be inclusive. Inclusion in name only can be viewed as tokenism, a policy of formally complying with efforts to achieve a goal by making small but insignificant gestures (*Merriam-Webster* 2014). The risk of tokenism is that Indigenous Pacific people are believed to be included and involved when the reality is they are even more invisible and that their issues continue to fall through the cracks. If any organization or group wants to be inclusive of Indigenous Pacific people, then the inclusion must be genuine and efforts must be made to ensure that Indigenous Pacific people are respectfully involved in all aspects of business and activities. This may mean that special efforts to build participation will be required to make the inclusion genuine.

In recognition of the special and unique relationships that all of these Indigenous populations have with the federal government, the secretary of the Department of Health and Human Services (DHHS 2005) has identified all of these groups as having "standing" for consultation within the Department of Health and Human Services, described previously.

## VOICES FROM THE COMMUNITY

In the following sections two of the co-authors, an Indigenous Pacific community leader and an Indigenous Pacific researcher, provide their perspective of the research process. Joey Quenga is the executive director of the Toa Institute, a community-based service organization. Dr. Raynald Samoa is an endocrinologist and community leader; he discusses the pros and cons of serving in the role of the Indigenous Pacific research scientist. Their perspective brings attention to the challenges a community leader faces and the strengths that position can bring with a focus on strong networks, accountability, community leadership, and benefits of the research to the community.

### Perspective: Indigenous Pacific Community Leader in Service to the Community

Like many minority community leaders, Indigenous Pacific community leaders are required to wear many different hats. In addition to the standard responsibilities required for running and maintaining a professional position, an Indigenous Pacific community leader carries many additional cultural and political duties to ensure all aspects of the community needs are met. For example, the Toa Institute Executive Director, Joey Quenga, is often called to give a blessing for a conference, visit Chamoru patients who have been flown from Guam to the United States for medical treatment (a 20-hour flight across the International Dateline), and travel to Washington, DC, to sing traditional songs for the congresswoman of Guam. These duties expand the standard workweek well beyond 40 hours and require a level of commitment and accountability that is expected by the Indigenous Pacific community.

Research with Indigenous Pacific communities must, at minimum, follow the general CBPR approach, including basic principles such as shared decision-making, equitable distribution of resources, and mutual benefit. In addition, there are a number of key issues that all researchers, both within the community and from outside the community, need to take into consideration when working with Indigenous Pacific people.

Researchers must be able to build rapport and become aware of key leaders in the community. Without these individuals, successful research may not be possible. It is, however, the responsibility of the researchers to understand that the reasons these individuals are leaders in their respective communities can also be the reasons that objectives may take longer than initially expected. Indigenous Pacific community leaders are responsible for ensuring that resources are available to meet the community's needs. The challenge for researchers is to understand that although community leaders understand the importance and long-term benefits of a properly executed research project, they must balance future needs with current needs. Focusing on one more than the other would be detrimental to any leader in the community and cause for distrust, having an adverse effect on participation in any potential research projects.

A leader in the Chomoru community instinctively seeks to protect the community with a warrior-like mentality. What are researchers thinking when they commit such energy and effort for a year or two and then just leave with no sense of responsibility to the community? Understanding how researchers can have an enormous impact on the people, it is the leader's role to pick and choose research projects carefully. This is a role that is taken seriously, and although resources are very limited, it is imperative that the community does not just "follow the funding."

While some researchers put an emphasis on projects for personal gain, such as advances in career, academic tenure, and publication, community leaders are not held to the same rules and regulations. It is not necessary to publish an article in order to be a community leader. Chomoru ancestors and community elders would rather the leaders "tend the land" than strive for academic tenure.

This is what is important to the Chomoru people. Any researcher who truly has the best interest of the community at heart should be prepared for many nights of one-on-one conversations, extensive meals with families, some manual labor, and the provision of much needed resources to the community.

Communities view academic and research institutions as resources that will lead to much-needed services in the underrepresented Indigenous Pacific community. If a study or research does not benefit the community, it is highly unlikely that the community will participate in future studies. Thus, it is the responsibility of the community leaders to have a grasp of the proposed study, understand the benefits and risks to the community, and, if accepted, present the study to the community in order to secure participation. Unfortunately, there are some researchers who do not fully comprehend the depth of responsibility required of a community leader and only see a partner that does not always make deadlines or is disinterested in editing publications. It is fortunate to partner with responsible researchers and educational institutions but there is a fine balance between being a community leader and trying to fill the goals of a research grant. Understanding the taboos of the culture and having the ability to inquire about subjects in a culturally sensitive manner is crucial for a successful study.

When conducting research with Indigenous Pacific people, it is important to understand that although cultures can be very diverse among Polynesians, Micronesians, and Melanesians, the entire Pacific Island community is aware of the importance of working with one another. It is this dependency between the different island communities that can make or break the reputation of a researcher. For example, when someone works with the Chamoru community, the work and how the researcher conducts business will be shared with the Samoan community who, in turn, will share with the Native Hawaiians and the Tongans.

In terms of resources, it is this spirit of collaboration that Indigenous Pacific communities must adhere to in order to secure particular grants or research projects. The Indigenous Pacific community is often called upon to partner with Asian/Pacific Islander organizations for specific projects and must be inclusive of the Asian community. In instances where there may be opportunity for resources to be directed to NHOPI individuals, efforts must be made to work in partnership, not in competition. The ability to adjust and be inclusive of many different communities is the reality of conducting research with these communities.

## Perspective: Indigenous Pacific Researcher Working With the Community

Conducting research in Indigenous Pacific communities can be extremely rewarding and at the same time exceedingly difficult. Research is viewed as a side attraction that community-based organizations (CBOs) are often pulled into without fully understanding the complexity of the process. The current landscape is made up of community leaders that have a strong interest in research motivated by short- and long-term gains for Indigenous Pacific communities and their representative organizations. The Indigenous Pacific community is faced with a number of major obstacles (limitations in study design development, grant writing, and protocol implementation when working with the community), which stem from a lack of the necessary skill capacity and not a lack of interest in collaborating on projects. Community leaders are generally from non–health-research backgrounds that traditionally entrusted outside investigators to ensure that the welfare of their communities was protected during a research study. The historical abuse of these relationships has prompted leaders to advocate for a more equal role in conducting research in their communities, resulting in a call for more community-academic partnerships that provide a more co-equal research relationship. As a result, this has provided more funding announcements promoting CBPR. As the appeal to form these relationships has increased, efforts to improve the needed skill set of these CBOs to conduct research in order to be equal partners in the research process are lacking. It often falls upon academic investigators to educate community researchers on good business practices, all aspects of study development, and grant writing to ensure a co-equal environment. This has proven to be a timely process that in turn obstructs grant application efforts when there is little time to formulate an application for submission. Thus, small, short-term projects have few associated long-term benefits when one considers the amount of time and resources needed to implement them.

The differences in backgrounds of academic and community investigators almost make a collaborative project a nearly insurmountable feat to accomplish. Through concentrating on similarities with partners in the community, projects have been mutually productive. CBO leaders are usually called to activism through indignities that they have either experienced or witnessed by being members of their communities. Thus, they have organized to fight for social justice and equity for their communities. Health disparities faced by the community and projects that aid in understanding or intervening with the long-term goal of rectifying those disparities are of interest to both the researcher and the community. This intertwined common interest has formed a foundation based on working towards equity through research. Thus, short-term projects should be developed with a long-term vision that provides not only a co-equal environment but a co-learning one as well. It should be noted that this approach takes a firm commitment to the philosophy that the investment placed into educating the community on how to conduct meaningful research will benefit the researcher's efforts for the entire duration of his or her research career.

### Protecting the Community

As discussed in Chapter 3 with regard to AIAN communities, Hawaiian and Indigenous Pacific communities may also utilize their own institutional review boards (IRBs). Papa Ola Lokahi, the Native Hawaiian Health Board, has an IRB which serves the Native Hawaiian Health Care Systems (NHHCS) and has the mission and purpose of maximizing benefits and minimizing risks of research among Native Hawaiian individuals and communities. It has the additional charge of educating researchers and building capacity within communities so that they can participate in research projects as partners to address community health concerns. The Native Hawaiian IRB was established because existing IRBs were lacking in awareness of potential harms to Native Hawaiian communities and were not appropriately addressing the needs of the NHHCS. Ongoing and rigorous training is provided for all the members, and the opinions and concerns of community members are as respected on the same level as that of the scientists and health professionals on the board.

## TAKE-HOME MESSAGES

Designing a meaningful research proposal is imperative for numerous reasons. The first is related to the severity of health disparities among Indigenous Pacific people. Indigenous Pacific people are facing disease epidemics and cannot afford to focus on issues that will not benefit their communities. Second, Indigenous Pacific people experience constant political threats, from the denial of federal recognition for Native Hawaiians, to the challenging of Native Hawaiian trust education (Kamehameha Schools), to the threat of nonrenewal of federal funding. These assaults are contemporary examples of facts, not speculations. Producing quality, meaningful research for Indigenous Pacific people demands that efforts to accurately describe the burden of disease and advocate for continued efforts to reduce that burden must be supported and promoted.

Third, conducting meaningful research in Indigenous Pacific people contributes to the compilation of accurate, documented scientific knowledge on their health. Recent studies have shown that racial misclassification in mortality data is as high as 72% in some minority communities (Arias et al. 2008). Effective and meaningful research can assist in identifying the true rate of disease and correct the inaccuracies reported in health statistics.

Fourth, conducting meaningful research in Indigenous Pacific people helps to restore trust and provide a framework for communities to effectively plan and grow. Though complicated and emotionally charged, the damage of cultural trauma in Indigenous communities may be soothed by addressing health disparities and improving the physical, emotional, and spiritual well-being of these communities through true community-based participatory strategies. By seeking to heal some of the pain and suffering caused by past wrongful research practices, perhaps the link between research and Indigenous populations might be strengthened.

The final message is to consider the analogy of comparing the role of researchers with the role of stars in navigation—just as seafaring ancestors utilized the stars to guide them in canoes in an effort to transfer resources from one island to another, so must researchers rely on community leaders to navigate in the communities. Indigenous Pacific communities recognize that there are researchers that understand the importance of being culturally competent, but it requires an investment in relationship building to understand the complexity of the community. The best way for Indigenous Pacific people to advance is to have the research come from the community, led by their own scientists, directed by their people. This way, the researchers are already familiar with cultural norms and can be held accountable for their actions. When this best practice isn't possible, the next best solution is to have the outside research team be guided and directed by the community.

## REFERENCES

Arias E, Schauman WS, Eschbach K, et al. 2008. The validity of race and Hispanic origin reporting on death certificates in the United States. *Vital Health Stat 2*. Oct 2008(148):1–23.

Berkley S, Titus D. 2009. *Berkley, Titus Urge White House to End Bush-Era Directives Against Travel to Las Vegas, Other Destinations*. Available at: http://votesmart.org/ public-statement/443696/berkley-titus-urge-white-house-to-end-bush-era-directives-against-travel-to-las-vegas-other-destinations#.UVYKslB6fIk. Accessed March 28, 2013.

Ghosh C. 2003. Healthy People 2010 and Asian Americans/Pacific Islanders: defining a baseline of information. *Am J Public Health*. 93(12):2093–2098.

Hawai'i Tourism Authority. 2013. *Annual Visitor Research*. Available at: http://www. hawaiitourismauthority.org/research/reports/annual-visitor-research. Accessed March 28, 2013.

Hirokawa R, Huang T, Pobutsky A, Nogues M, Salvail F, Nguyen HD. 2004. Hawaii diabetes report. Hawaii: Hawaii State Department of Health.

Hoyert DL, Kung HC. 1997. Asian or Pacific Islander mortality, Selected States, 1992. *Mon Vit Stat Rep*. 46(1 Suppl). Hyattsville, Maryland: National Center for Health Statistics.

Indian Health Care Improvement Act. P.L. 93-644.

Keighley E, Quested C, Mccuddin C, et al. 2007. Nutrition and health in modernizing Samoans: temporal trends and adaptive perspectives, in health change in the Asia-Pacific region. In: Ulijaszek SJ, Ohtsuka R, editors. *Biocultural and Epidemiological Approaches*. Cambridge, MA: Cambridge University Press. p. 147–191.

Merriam-Webster.com. Available at: http://www.merriam-webster.com/dictionary/ tokenism. Accessed July 27, 2013.

Minton N, Silva NK, editors. 1998. *Kue: The Hui Aloha Aina Anti-Annexation Petitions, 1897–1898*. Available at: http://libweb.hawaii.edu/digicoll/annexation/petition.html. Accessed July 16, 2013.

*Native American Programs Act of 1974.* P.L. 93-638, as amended. *Indian Health Care Improvement Act.* P.L. 93-644.

Office of Management and Budget Federal Register Notice of October 30, 1997. 62 FR 58782–58790.

Ponce N, Tseng W, Ong P, et al. 2009. *The State of Asian American, Native Hawaiian and Pacific Islander Health in California Report.* Prepared for the Honorable Mike Eng, Assemblymember, 49th Assembly District. Sacramento, CA. Available at: http://www. cdph.ca.gov/programs/Documents/AANHPI_report_April2009.pdf. Accessed July 16, 2013.

Rush EC, Freitas I, Plank LD. 2009. Body size, body composition and fat distribution: comparative analysis of European, Maori, Pacific Island and Asian Indian adults. *Br J Nutr.* 2009;102(4):632–41.

Spoehr H. 2006. *Threads in the Human Tapestry: The Disaggregation of the API Identifier and the Importance of Having the NHOPI (Native Hawaiian and Other Pacific Islander) Category in Data Collection, Analysis, and Reporting.* Honolulu, HI: Papa Ola Lokahi.

Taualii M. 2007. Self-rated health status comparing Pacific Islanders to Asians. *J Health Disparities Res Pract.* 1(2): Article 7. Available at: http://digitalscholarship.unlv.edu/jhdrp/vol1/iss2/7. Accessed September 28, 2013.

US Census Bureau. 2010. Census of Population, Public Law 94-171 Redistricting Data File.

US Code Title 20, Chapter 3, Subchapter XIII, § 80q-14. 2011. Available at: http://www. gpo.gov/fdsys/pkg/USCODE-2011-title20/html/USCODE-2011-title20.htm. Accessed July 21, 2013.

US Department of Health and Human Services. 2005. Department Tribal Consultation Policy. Available at: http://www.hhs.gov/iea/tribal/tribalconsultation/hhs-consultation-policy.pdf. Accessed July 27, 2013.

**6**

---

# Successful Approaches to Research Through Collaborative Design and Culturally Relevant Methods

Felicia Schanche Hodge, DrPH, and Roxanne Struthers, RN, PhD, CHTP, AHN-BC, CTN

## INTRODUCTION

The American Indian (AI) population is one of the most researched groups in the nation (Crazy Bull 1997). Decades of research experiences have taught numerous and agonizing lessons to American Indian and Alaska Native peoples. These experiences resulted in significant barriers to research initiatives. At the same time, these experiences created the impetus for more acceptable, adaptable, and culturally sensitive methods and approaches.

This chapter explores lessons learned while conducting research among AI populations. The importance of defining the problem, finding culturally appropriate approaches, reciprocating in the research process, and disseminating research findings are discussed as part of the research participatory experience. The research skills and experiences of the research team combined with understanding and integrating AI cultural methods of education, training, and interaction as well as resources of the community can provide a more acceptable and amenable research experience.

As more researchers experience positive and successful investigations, it is important to share lessons gained from these studies with others. It is not uncommon for researchers to experience similar problems during or following a research event. Misunderstandings can stall a project and even lead to errors in implementing the research protocol. Differences in languages, word construction, and expectations can influence the interpretation of instructions. If a summer social gathering, such as a powwow, is always attended by community members, survey takers or study subjects may drop all project work to attend cultural events, with little or no understanding of the impact a breach in protocol time frames may have on the project. It is important to obtain information on all possible special events, interferences, and past experiences that may have an impact on the conduct of the study. This process may come easier to a Native researcher and may be facilitated through a community key informant or "gatekeeper." The experiences of successful researchers are invaluable for all researchers, and may make or break a project. Following are descriptions of research projects conducted among various tribes that illustrate lessons learned and enable a discussion of successful research approaches and methodologies.

## DEFINING THE RESEARCH PROJECT

### Identifying the Problem

Identifying the problem or issues to be examined is a significant first step in research. For example, in 1989 the National Cancer Institute supported and funded a collaboration of cancer research projects targeting American Indians, Alaska Natives, and Native Hawaiians in various sites across the United States (Hodge and Glover 1999). These projects utilized various approaches to identify the problem, design the methodology, and implement the programs. Hodge et al. (1995) partnered with 18 California tribes in the initial formative stages to identify the priority areas for research. Tribes were asked via written correspondence to provide input as to what subject matter was considered important and desirable for research. Cigarette smoking was selected as a significant concern for research intervention and a participatory process was modeled utilizing an all-Indian advisory board, focus groups, and community input in the development of the survey. Problem areas were discussed freely and worked out to mutual satisfaction between the researchers and the tribe/

community. This example demonstrates that once the problem area is identified and agreed upon, all parties can move forward knowing the scope of the study and exploration.

## Study Participants

Research can be described as a systematic approach to discovery or knowledge. A key function of research is the identification of data sources, collection of data, analysis of findings, and reporting of research finding. The failure of many researchers to collect data from participants, resulting from poor recruitment or high attrition, is not an uncommon phenomenon during the research process. Poor recruitment of minority participants in clinical trials has been documented and discussed by Native researchers (Spilker and Cramer 1992, Hodge et al. 2000, Bloom et al. 1991, Hodge and Casken 1999, Hodge and Stubbs 1999, Hodge 2003). Understanding that failure to recruit and retain study participants stems from historical events helps researchers recognize and address the issue. Years of data collection by the federal government, health agencies, special censuses, and anthropologists and other researchers caused distrust toward researchers. Filling out reams of questionnaires with little or no understanding or explanation causes frustration, exasperation, and annoyance when people are presented with yet one more document to complete. Numerous forms with questions on marital status, income, health problems, feelings, and attitudes may seem even more invasive, and sometimes study participants find the questions offensive or simply incomprehensible. This can result in an incomplete questionnaire or refusal to continue with the study. In some instances, research has actually harmed or caused the stigmatization of AI peoples and communities, causing further animosity (Davis and Reid 1999). Community input while developing the survey, using focus groups and pilot testing of the survey, and employing American Indians as research assistants to administer the survey can help alleviate obstacles in these situations.

## Measures or Tools

Defining a problem leads to designing questions to be asked, as well as the research tools used to measure the problem. Utilizing appropriate research tools is vital to obtaining accurate measures. A questionnaire that is inappropriate, difficult to complete, or not completely understandable will prevent many participants from responding, responding truthfully, or continuing in the study, or it may impede the degree of understanding or knowledge obtained from the participant. Often, standardized tests that measure such constructs as depression, social support, wellness, and quality of life may not be applicable to American Indians in research situations. For instance, the CES-D (Centers for Epidemiology Studies–Depression) scale has been used to measure depressive symptomology for a number of years. Validated among an elderly group of White females in Montana, this scale has been met with much consternation among some tribal groups (Radloff 1977). Usability may be compromised by questions regarding historic and cultural influence on scale item definitions (Hodge and Kipnis 1995).

Successful methods of measuring social support in a community or among individuals vary by ethnicity. Researchers have measured social support among the Black community in a breast cancer study through the use of church attendance (Bloom et al. 1991). Hodge and Casken (1999) have used a measure of friends and family members in a scale to measure social support among American Indians. This is justified because relationships with friends and family described by many Natives are often comingled. Small, isolated reservations may indeed result in one's friend being a cousin, sibling, or other relative.

Measuring such concepts as wellness and quality of life are more complex. Many tribes view illness as a cultural construct, with varying explanations and ceremonies to treat the illness. Being out of balance and out of harmony is a common view of illness. Taboos, witchcraft, and historic traumas may also be included in the view of illness. The value of wealth (income), education, and perception of status is often viewed quite differently in Indian country. Investigation is needed into Native community differences in response to pain, fatalism, and the meaning of life. The goals of a community, the magnitude of culture, and the explanation of problems and issues need clarification when conducting research in these communities.

## COMMUNITY-BASED PARTICIPATORY RESEARCH

Community-based participatory research (CBPR) is a process that encourages communities to participate in the development, implementation and evaluation of research (Minkler 2005, Trimble et al. 2010). This process has encountered difficulties in AI communities. Inequalities in power, perceptions, and definitions of research terms contribute to incompatible academic-community discussions. Mohatt and Thomas (2005) emphasize the need for researchers to understand the influence of culture in the formulation of research questions, methods, and interpretation. The following are key challenges discussed by a number of authors (Wallerstein and Duran 2009, Fisher and Ball 2003, Fisher and Ball 2005, Christopher 2005) for American Indians as equal partners in the CBPR process:

- translating research findings to populations who have high variability in culture and resources;
- listening to and incorporating cultural practices, beliefs, and theories;
- translating language;
- control of the research process by academics;
- insufficient attention to implementation within the organizational culture; and
- lack of trust between researchers and underrepresented communities.

Use of such research terms as *institutionalization* or *collaborators* may trigger resistance and historical memories of assimilationist policies or betrayal. Additionally, terms such as *control* and *contamination* may result in resistance by the community.

CBPR, as operationalized by AI communities, means that tribes are equal partners, participating fully in the identification of the problem, the research design, and the selection of measures, participants, and findings. As American Indians are a collective society whose decisions are made by the group or by elders, and not on an individual basis, this dynamic is an important cultural process to consider in designing research.

Community involvement in research can present in several forms: partnerships, contracts or consultancy with tribal advisory councils, and tribal council stewardship. Indeed, tribes are beginning to assert ownership over research data, voice their interpretation of research findings, and control publications by guiding publication topics and having the authority to approve or disapprove publications. Ensuring that interpretation of the research data reflects the tribal culture and that value-laden measures are not used or reported is an important function of tribal institutional review boards (IRBs) and advisory boards. In addition, many tribes are starting to require that research teams provide training workshops or meetings in the tribal community prior, during, and after the research (Maldonado 2005, Navajo Human Research Review Board 2007). These workshops provide some interaction with the community and help to educate members on various research topics. Videos and publications on the history of the tribe or the urban community may be exchanged so that the research team can expand their knowledge and understanding of the tribal culture and community.

## CULTURALLY APPROPRIATE APPROACHES

### Talking Circles

The *talking circle* is a well-known method of intragroup communication in many Indian communities (Hodge et al. 1996). There are several types of circles that have been used for communication, problem solving, and healing. The most common of circles is the "sharing" group, in which people gather to discuss issues and share information and news events. There is no organization of the group, no format or theme, just a method of forming a circle group for communication. The second circle grouping is somewhat more formal, constructed for groups who gather together to solve problems and to mediate disagreement. These talking circles allow for the airing of problems or issues and provide the opportunity for participants to hear and to be heard. All parties are encouraged to speak and come to some resolution. Facilitators guide the process so that all can speak. A third circle is the healing circle, guided by a facilitator with the goal of guiding the participants to increased knowledge, group support, and insight designed to improve lifestyle behaviors and reduce risky behaviors.

Several projects have successfully utilized talking circles in cancer control, wellness, and diabetes intervention (Hodge and Stubbs 1999, Hodge 2003). Similar to the Hawaiian *kokua* groups (the concept of kokua is defined as a mutual willingness to assist without an expectation or return and without having to be asked), the talking circles model employs the concept of group support, a comfortable and safe environment, and the use of traditional Native ways of respect, resources, knowledge, and insight (Hodge and Stubbs 1999, Banner et al. 1999). Struthers et al. (2003) describe the processes as follows:

> At the beginning of each circle, the meeting area was cleansed and purified with sage (a traditional herb). A prayer was said by one of the Talking Circle

participants 'over the food, over what we are doing ...and the positive things that come out of it.' Tobacco, along with a plate of food served at the Talking Circle meal, was offered to the spirits/creator. The curriculum itself comprised Western explanations and presented diabetes as a disease entity. During the course of the Talking Circles sessions, however, values of American Indian culture began to percolate through the Western material in the form of dialogue, exchanges, and responses to the curriculum. Humor was much in evidence, as well as respect for the opinions of all, and the ability to 'talk about a lot of things...to talk about the culture... [and] ...wanting to be well for the future of our children.' These strategies assured that a bond and connection, very important in Indian culture, was formed between the facilitator and the participants. 'The circles bonded them (participants) closer...The Talking Circles participants are doing more stuff together than before...And even after they (the circles) are over...it's like they're still linked together somehow...Mainly the bonding strength of knowing they're not the only ones dealing with this (diabetes).'

A talking circle is commonly composed of 15 to 20 members who meet periodically to share information, support each other, and offer solutions to problems. This technique is historically important to tribal communication for sharing and problem solving. Often, following an opening of the session with a story and presentation of the education material, an arrow or feather is passed around the circle of participants signifying individual control of the floor. When talking or sharing, each participant has complete control of the floor without interruption, while other participants attentively listen. Passing on the talisman signifies passing the authority to speak to the nextvparticipant. The format of the talking circle allows each participant to discuss his or her fears, concerns, or needs in relation to the subject matter in an acceptable, comfortable, and safe manner. Meeting in a circle also ensures shared equality and that all voices will be heard. Maintaining confidentially, respect, and learning the presented lesson are important aspects of the circles.

In the above manner, the talking circle should not be mistaken for a focus group. Focus groups are formed to elicit information from participants. Although similarities between both techniques include the gathering of group members and encouraging the sharing and talking among the group (particularly the answering of key questions), the purpose and outcome of the focus groups centers on the identification and gathering of information for other reasons. The gathering of information, members likes and dislikes, as well the garnering of better understanding of the perception and the behaviors of a group are at the core of focus groups. Talking circles, on the other hand, are structured to enhance communication within a group.

Caution is advised not to use the talking circle in a negative or a controlling fashion. The technique to the talking circle is to enhance the learning environment—not to force change or to shame, cajole, or reveal "secrets" of others. The talking circle technique encourages; it does not force or require participation.

## Storytelling

The use of storytelling as a culturally appropriate approach to education has been used successfully in several intervention research projects (Hodge and Stubbs 1999, Hodge 2003, Tooze 1959, Hodge et al. 2002). American Indian culture has traditionally been passed on through the use of oral narrative. It is a spoken culture, with a rich oral tradition. Language gives meaning and life to traditions through the telling of stories that pass from generation to generation. These stories, sometimes called legends or myths, have been told for thousands of years and are still being told and retold, reshaped and refitted to meet their audience's changing needs, or even created anew to fit contemporary situations and visions.

The traditional stories told during the course of the talking circles transcend tribal boundaries, as they emphasize values significant to all Indian tribes. These stories nurture the culture and provide positive incentives for health promotion and prevention. Such a cultural approach to wellness is readily applicable to all tribes, since the use of storytelling to relay important messages and to provide positive direction is a common tribal tradition. Using the talking circle and AI traditional stories provides a culturally sensitive base for the presentation of an educational curriculum and has been useful in behavior change interventions (diet and nutrition, physical activity, weight loss), projects to increase knowledge (diabetes, cancer, tobacco control), and general healthcare intervention models (Hodge and Stubbs 1999, Hodge et al. 1996, Struthers et al. 2003, Hodge et al. 2002).

Storytelling is a common method of communication, pedagogy, and entertainment among American Indians. Employing storytelling to gather research data helps to build trust, expands the opportunity for participatory research, and utilizes an acceptable Indigenous method in the process of research. Several reports of research misuse and abuse has created distrust of researchers in AI communities (Wilson and Yellow Bird 2005, Smith 1999). The use of narrative stories may help to counteract this, as participation in storytelling is an honorable occasion, one in which the process of storytelling encourages the engagement of key informants.

The opportunity for researchers to better understand such constructs as etiology, treatment expectations, and experiences formed by the storyteller's words places the storyteller and the researcher in a unique situation. The storyteller is in control of the research process, in terms of areas of explorations, value of the terms or explanations, and the process of imparting information. The researcher has an obligation to report on the study findings in order to present world views, illness beliefs, domain structures, and the meanings of cultural practices not always obvious in the narrative. It is critical that the researcher understands and reports on the process and the information, with which he or she has been provided, and does so within the unique social and historical contexts of these populations; for the storyteller tells more than just a story—that individual reports on the lived experiences, history, perceptions, and world views of a unique group of people.

## RECIPROCITY AND RESEARCH

The utilization of mutual resources in conducting research is another important area to consider. The concept of reciprocating in the research process has been discussed by Davis and Reid (1999):

> If researchers take something valuable, such as participant's ideas, time, or bodily fluids, then they must return something of equal value, such as skills, employment, training, mentoring, or increased access to funding.

The days of "helicopter" research (dropping into communities, obtaining research data, and flying out without leaving anything behind) is unacceptable. Examining how the research will truly benefit the community is recommended when using a research process that is participatory so that harm will not come to the participants or to the community. Additionally, researchers need to be cognizant of the need to maintain good relationships with the tribes. That particular failure in the research experience has long-lasting repercussions, locally as well as nationally.

## Building Social Capital

A participatory process continuously utilizes resources of the community to help maximize efficiency, cultural acceptability, and trust. The concept of social capital encompasses features of social life—networks, norms, and trust—which enable participants to work in concert more efficiently to effectuate desired outcomes (Putnam 1995). In AI communities these resources may include community manpower, language, educational methods, formal and informal leadership, and the ideal of collective community. Tapping into the local manpower pool to hire and train research staff has provided much needed employment on reservations. Another benefit is the provision of training and education in a culturally acceptable manner. Several talking circles research projects have employed and trained local Native staff to organize the circles, recruit and engage the participants, present the curriculum, and guide the discussion. These local lay health personnel (also known as lay health workers, lay health advisors, lay health educators, peer educators, and community health workers) are utilized in the community to provide education to peers and to perform other tasks. Responsibilities include serving as cultural mediators and links between minority people and health agencies, helping to establish social networks, offering social support, mobilizing community health resources, providing health knowledge, and improving the quality of healthcare through continuous utilization of services (Hodge and Glover 1999, Eng and Smith 1995, Digan et al. 1998, Witmer et al. 1995).

## Peer Facilitators

The concept of working with the community and of using community resources are important aspects of several studies (Hodge et al. 2000, Hodge and Stubbs 1999, Hodge 2003, Struthers et al. 2003). Peer facilitators act as interpreters and liaisons to the local community. They are excellent resources and serve as sounding boards and provide direction in relations with the community. In a study of diabetes among the Sioux and Winnebago, peer facilitators were trained on all aspects of diabetes relative to prevention, treatment, nonadherence to treatment, the disease process, and control. They proved to be excellent interpreters to the study participants, providing information in a format and with words that were readily understandable to the study participants. The information was presented in a cultural context, which resulted in a higher acceptance and adoption of recommended behaviors (Struthers et al. 2003). The congruence of the peer facilitators and the culture of the community acted to reinforce the acceptance and adoption of the interventions. Lay health workers are well equipped to act as intermediaries between the cultures of the mainstream and the target culture. The ability to interpret and communicate often-complex Western medical knowledge on prevention and treatment of disease to AI community members who live in rural, remote, underserved reservations is invaluable.

## DISSEMINATION OF RESEARCH FINDINGS

Publication in peer-reviewed journals is an important and necessary process for career development and tenure in academic institutions. Even so, the publication of research findings is another area in which the community must be engaged and negotiation may be necessary. Tribes may require a preview of publications and desire the liberty to make recommendations to assure that nothing offensive or misleading is reported. It is important as well that tribes be sure that their culture is portrayed in an appropriate and accurate manner, and that tribal sovereignty is protected. Issues of confidentiality are also of concern, as small communities or tribal members can potentially be identified by demographic variables or by illness categories. These problems have been dealt with through conducting pre-publication review with community or tribal leaders, placing tribal research staff or partners as contributors on publications, and obtaining tribal approval for publication. Publication may be planned for lay or community reports, tribal council reports, or scientific journal articles. Publication drafts can be disseminated to tribal councils or to tribal IRBs. It is important to provide sufficient time for these committees or boards to review and respond to the article. Unfortunately, many of these groups meet infrequently or sporadically. Maintaining good relationships with a gatekeeper and presenting the publication orally and in writing provides the opportunity for tribal groups to ask pertinent questions in a timely manner.

Submitting copies of final publications to the tribe and all relevant staff and groups is also highly recommended.

## SUMMARY

Reviewing lessons learned and successful approaches and methods for conducting research among AI populations is important to Indian and non-Indian researchers interested in pursuing research among these groups. Approaching AI communities and actually asking for input to identify the research problem and the best way to gather information, select measurement tools and data collection, and work with the assets of the community, provides for a culturally appropriate approach to research. The examples presented in this chapter highlight methods employed to ensure success of the research process. These successes center on the concept of social capital—utilizing the resources of the community or population to better realize positive outcomes. This can only be accomplished through a collaborative research process. The research skills and experiences of the research team, combined with understanding and integrating AI cultural methods of education, training, and interaction as well as the resources of the community, can provide a more acceptable and amenable research experience.

## REFERENCES

Banner RO, Gotay CC, Enos R, et al. 1999. Effects of a culturally tailored intervention to increase breast and cervical cancer screening in Native Hawaiians. In: Glover C, Hodge FS, editors. *Native Outreach: A Report to American Indian, Alaska Native and Native Hawaiian Communities.* Washington, DC: National Institutes of Health. pp. 98–139.

Bloom JR, Grazier K, Hodge F, et al. 1991. Factors affecting the use of screening mammography among African American women. *Cancer Epidemiol Biomarkers Prev.* 1(1):75–82.

Christopher S. 2005. Recommendations for conducting successful research with Native Americans. *J Cancer Educ.* 20(1 suppl):47–51.

Crazy Bull C. 1997. A Native conversation about research and scholarship. *Tribal College: J Am Indian Higher Educ.* 9(1):17–23.

Davis S, Reid R. 1999. Practicing participatory research in American Indian communities. *Am J Clin Nutr.* 69:755S–759S.

Digan MB, Michielutte R, Wells HB, et al. 1998. Health education to increase screening for cervical cancer among Lumbee Indian women in North Carolina. *Health Educ Res.* 13(4):545–556.

Eng E, Smith J. 1995. Natural helping functions of lay health advisors in breast cancer education. *Breast Cancer Res Treat.* 35(1):23–29.

Fisher PA, Ball TJ. 2003. Tribal participatory research: Mechanisms of a collaborative model. *Am J Community Psychol.* 32(3/4):207–216.

Fisher PA, Ball TJ. 2005. Balancing empiricism and local cultural knowledge in the design of prevention research. *J Urban Health.* 82:(2 Suppl. 3) iii44–iii55.

Hodge FS. 2003. *Wellness Circles: An American Indian approach.* (Grant No. R01 NR04722, 6/1/98–8/30/03). Bethesda, MD: National Institutes of Health, National Institute for Nursing Research.

Hodge FS, Casken J. 1999. American Indian breast cancer project: educational development and implementation. *Am Indian Cult Res J.* 23(3):113–118.

Hodge FS, Cummings S, Kipnis P, et al. 1995. Prevalence of smoking among adult American Indian clinic users in northern California. *Prev Med.* 24:441–446.

Hodge FS, Fredericks L, Rodriguez B. 1996. American Indian women's talking circle: a cervical cancer screening and prevention project. *Cancer.* 78(7):1592–1597.

Hodge FS, Glover C. 1999. The National Cancer Institute's research efforts in Native American communities: approaches used and lessons learned. *Native Outreach: A Report to American Indian, Alaska Native and Native Hawaiian communities.* Washington DC: National Institutes of Health. pp. 102–111.

Hodge FS, Kipnis P. 1995. Demoralization: a useful concept for case management with Native Americans. In: Manolas P, editor. *The Cross-Cultural Practice of Critical Case Management in Mental Health.* New York, NY: Haworth Press.

Hodge FS, Pasqua A, Marquez CA, et al. 2002. Utilizing traditional storytelling to promote wellness in American Indian communities. *J Transcult Nurs.* 13(1):6–11.

Hodge FS, Stubbs H. 1999. Talking circles: Increasing cancer knowledge among American Indian women. *Cancer Res Therapy.* 8:103–111.

Hodge FS, Weinmann S, Roubideaux Y. 2000. Recruitment of American Indians and Alaska Natives into clinical trials. *Ann Epidemiol.* 10(8):S41–S48.

Maldonado R. 2005. *Navajo Nation IRB/Research Protocols.* The Native Peoples Technical Assistance Office. Window Rock, AZ: Historic Preservation Department, Cultural Resource Compliance Section.

Minkler M. 2005. Community-based research partnerships: challenges and opportunities. *J Urban Health.* 82:ii3–12.

Mohatt GV, Thomas LR. 2005. I wonder, why would you do it that way? Ethical dilemmas in doing participatory research with Alaska Native communities. In: Trimble JE, Fisher CB, editors. *The Handbook of Ethical Research with Ethnocultural Populations & Communities.* Thousand Oaks, CA: Sage Publications. pp. 93–114.

Navajo Human Research Review Board. 2007. *IRB Research Protocol Application Guidelines.* Window Rock, AZ: Navajo Division of Health.

Putnam RD. 1995. Tuning in, tuning out: the strange disappearance of social capital in America. *Political Sci Politics.* 28:664–683.

Radloff LS. 1977. The CES-D scale: a self-report depression scale for research in the general population. *Appl Psychol Measurement.* 1:385–401.

Smith LT. 1999. *Decolonizing Methodologies: Research and Indigenous Peoples.* New York, NY: Palgrave Macmillan.

Spilker B, Cramer JA. 1992. *Patient Recruitment in Clinical Trials.* New York, NY: Raven Press.

Struthers R, Hodge FS, De Cora L, et al. 2003. The experience of Native peer facilitators in the campaign against Type 2 diabetes. *J Rural Health.* 19(2):174–180.

Tooze R.1959. *Storytelling.* Upper Saddle River, New Jersey: Prentice-Hall, Inc.

Trimble JE, Scharron-del Rio MR, Bernal G. 2010. The itinerant researcher: ethical and methodological issues in conducting cross-cultural mental health research. In: Jack DC, Ali A, editors. *Silencing the Self Across Cultures. Depression and Gender in the Social World.* New York, NY: Oxford University Press.

Wallerstein N, Duran B. 2010. Community-based participatory research contributions to intervention research: the intersection of science and practice to improve health equity. *Am J Public Health.* 100 (supp 1):S40–S46.

Wilson WA, Yellow Bird M. 2005. *For Indigenous Eyes Only: A Decolonization Handbook.* Santa Fe, NM: School of American Research Press.

Witmer AS, Finocchio SL, Leslie J, et al. 1995. Community health workers: integral members of the health care work force. *Am J Public Health.* 85(8):1055–1058.

# 7

# Guidelines for Conducting Successful Community-Based Participatory Research in American Indian and Alaska Native Communities

Lillian Tom-Orme, RN, PhD, MPH, FAAN

## INTRODUCTION

Community-based participatory research (CBPR) is a relatively new phenomenon for American Indian/Alaska Native (AIAN) communities. It is defined as research generated collaboratively in a partnership between the scientific community and the population being studied, with benefits for both entities. It involves community representation in all phases and aspects of the study as a means of generating highly relevant findings that are ethical and beneficial (Aaron and Bass 2002). In the past, some researchers may have unknowingly exploited communities by emphasizing only the negative or pathological characteristics of communities. The goal of CBPR is to translate findings into comprehensive programs that improve the health of local populations by taking a positive approach to health and wellness through planned, coordinated, participatory, culturally competent, and ongoing efforts (Green and Mercer 2001).

The Tribal Preparatory Research (TPR) framework is a research method specifically focused on tribal communities with the understanding that they have experienced historical trauma that rendered them oppressed, discriminated against, and disempowered (Fisher and Ball 2003). The four mechanisms of TPR (tribal oversight, use of facilitator, training and employing community members, and application of culturally specific assessment and intervention methods) provide underlying principles that guide the relationship between researcher and community throughout the study process. The TPR process was derived from social science research, but could be adapted to public health or other disciplines. TPR emphasizes social change and community empowerment as an endpoint.

While CBPR has existed in community development, and in social, educational, and health delivery research, its recent reemergence in public health and clinical settings, particularly among ethnic minority communities, marks a new beginning in collaborative research. Medical and health practitioners have historically used a top-down approach based on the biomedical model that many view as paternalistic. The profession of nursing has been a leader in introducing a more collaborative approach between researcher and hospital staff and later between researcher and the community. Specifically, Leininger (1970, 2002), a nurse-anthropologist, founder of transcultural nursing, and theorist espoused anthropological approaches to gain the "emic" perspective (the informant's personal viewpoint) in health-illness situations through qualitative research. She developed these concepts and constructs into a transcultural health model called the Sunrise Model, which requires a global perspective and active community dialog in culturally competent research and care (Leininger 1970, Leininger and McFarland 2002).

Recently, health education and public health research have contributed to the evolution of CBPR into the widely accepted process and model in which we are now engaged, particularly in ethnic minority communities (Potvin et al. 2003, Wallerstein and Duran 2006). In Native or Indigenous CBPR, four principles have been identified for implementation in community programs (Potvin et al. 2003):

1. Equal partnership of community and researcher in all phases of a project,
2. Structural and functional integration of intervention and evaluation research components,

3. Flexibility in responding to demands of the broader environment, and
4. Inclusion of learning opportunities for all involved.

One of the many ways that ethnic communities began to increase discussion between communities and researchers involved a historic meeting on May 17, 1997. Former President Clinton made a formal apology to the surviving members of the 1932–1972 Tuskegee study and to the nation for the unethical and racist research that took place in the Tuskegee syphilis experiments (White House 1997). Several follow-up meetings took place to discuss ways that researchers could avoid making the same mistakes while being more inclusive of community needs in health-related research. This author was part of one of these meetings that included researchers from various communities of color. Subsequently, CBPR gained momentum in ethnic and Native communities during this period.

One such meeting in the American Indian community involved two dozen Native researchers and consumers who met with the National Institutes of Health (NIH) and the Indian Health Service (IHS) August 23–24, 1999. The purpose of the meeting was to identify American Indian research training needs and to develop recommendations about existing funding mechanisms and new programs (Kaufman and Associates, 1999, unpublished report). However, participants could not immediately identify these needs without also discussing barriers to research and research training. Among such issues discussed was the lack of trust and credibility that creates a schism between American Indian communities and researchers, especially in medical and health-related research. Recommendations to funding agencies included allowing more flexibility and time to plan a collaborative study and to obtain research approval, emphasizing capacity building in the local infrastructure, hiring and training students during the research process, and acknowledging that tribes are sovereign nations and may have different expectations than those of the standard research-intensive institutions or funding agencies.

## GROUNDING THE RESEARCH QUESTION IN THE COMMUNITY

In transcultural and public health research, the best type of community-based research occurs when both researcher and community agree on the most pressing health challenges and the most culturally appropriate and sound research design (Tom-Orme 2002a). Occasionally, researchers write a grant application that is funded without any contact or agreement on the part of the tribe or the local community. This approach is viewed as culturally insensitive by many tribal communities and highly likely to fail.

In an urban situation, a researcher must visit with the leaders or administrators of the social, education, or health program as well as participate in activities. Cultural immersion is an acceptable and preferred manner of being introduced to a community where local and shared practices dominate. Taking time to listen to stories is another immersion approach (Tom-Orme 2000). Holding focus groups, conducting sharing sessions, and attending community meetings are other ways to explore the need to modify research questions or methods.

In a reservation setting, cultural immersion is also important. The researcher should visit several times to acquaint his or herself with the life ways of the people; otherwise, one risks being seen as an outsider or "helicopter" researcher, as described in Chapter 6.

## RESPONDING TO COMMUNITY CONCERNS

Tribes may request researchers conduct a particular health promotion or disease prevention project in the community. A common practice is the tendency to focus only on the negative aspects of health issues or social structure. For instance, one might expound entirely on the negative social effects of alcoholism that then generalizes to the entire population, thereby painting a terribly dysfunctional picture of the tribe (Beauvais 1998, Beals et al. 2009). The positive factors or strengths of tribal communities are frequently overlooked but need to be acknowledged and reinforced as sustaining health practices (Tom-Orme 2002b). For example, American Indian women have been characterized as having a high rate of teen pregnancy, low education, late prenatal visits, and a tendency to smoke or use alcohol during pregnancy. But community strengths such as the support given to teen mothers through the matriarchal or matrilineal social and cultural clan system is easily overlooked because researchers may not know enough about the community to look for these important cultural norms or may simply not measure them.

Since the biomedical model focuses on searching for pathologic conditions, a sacred and important way of life is minimized. Tribal people value their young, as they are seen as the next generation to carry on their legacy, thus the concept of *the seventh generation.* (*Seven generations* is an ideology that embraces a conscious use of the Earth's resources, respectful treatment of others, and the responsibility of the current generation to those generations that will follow.) Babies receive blessings from community elders when they are given names or their socialization is celebrated through the First Laugh ceremony, a Navajo tradition of welcoming a baby into the world. These traditions ought to be interpreted as Indigenous health teachings that contribute to healthy communities. Carrese and Rhodes' (1995) qualitative study exemplifies the local community's insistence on avoiding negative thoughts or speech, focusing instead on the positives to create *hozho*, a Navajo philosophy of life and longevity.

Native communities are becoming more assertive and educated about research. Researchers need to be prepared to explain the following regarding their prospective studies in addition to the issues described in earlier chapters:

- The benefits to the community;
- The benefits to the individual;
- How findings will be reported and in what form, especially if they reflect negatively on the community;
- If interventions will be conducted to change or promote healthy behaviors;
- How questions about taboo words or culturally sensitive conditions will be addressed; and
- Potential policy implications of the study.

## AGREEING ON APPROPRIATE RESEARCH METHODS

Researchers need to take the time to thoroughly explain the research methods and procedures to tribal reviewers and the community. For example, what is the difference between retrospective and prospective studies? When is each type of study best used? Some tribes prefer a delayed control method in lieu of the traditional case-control or experimental study method so that all study participants benefit from an intervention. Focus groups followed by intervention studies have become popular among tribes over the past two decades (Tom-Orme 1991). In a focus group approach, study participants provide their unique perspectives about their experiences with a certain illness, state their concerns about various approaches previously used by researchers, or assist researchers in developing culturally appropriate research tools or designs. The focus group method can be advantageous and has several benefits for both researcher and community (Tom-Orme 1991, Strickland 1999). Unfortunately, some researchers may mistakenly believe that this is a quick way to collect information without investing the time and resources required of true participatory action research.

Clinical trials previously have not been well received, but now as tribes and AIAN individuals have more exposure to respectful researchers and are adequately informed about the benefits of research, confidence about enrolling in clinical trials is increasing (Kaur J, Roubideax M; personal correspondence; April 24, 2003). For example, cancer rates are increasing in some tribal communities, and personal experiences with cancer have varied depending on knowledge, awareness, and access to detection and treatment (Becker et al. 1993; Lanier et al. 2001; Hampton et al. 1996). Researchers who are sensitive to AIAN concerns about cancer treatment and healthcare situations are beginning to collaborate with cancer centers to bring cutting-edge technology and trials to Native communities (Petereit and Burhansstipanov 2008).

## NEGOTIATING COSTS AND BENEFITS TO PARTICIPANTS

Researchers conducting a study in a community need to consider budgeting for nontraditional items such as childcare, travel to and from the interview site, and other incentives for participation. Tribal communities frequently do not have drop-in childcare centers, thus participants may need childcare services during the time of their study interview or involvement. Often young mothers or grandmothers have small children to care for and therefore may be otherwise unable to participate.

Many times low-income Indian participants have to travel some distance to a central location to participate in a study. To encourage participation and give back to the community, researchers should provide a small incentive to participants, such as a grocery voucher, a gas card, a phone card, or small gift items such as a calendar, mug, t-shirt, or cash. Importantly, the amount of the gift or incentive should not be considered coercive but should provide appropriate compensation for the level of participation and the time required.

## WORKING WITH THE INSTITUTIONAL REVIEW BOARDS

Increasingly, tribes are developing their own institutional or human participants review board (IRB or HRB) or some type of tribal board to review and decide on studies for their tribe (American Indian Law Center 1999). The Navajo Nation probably has the most elaborate and complex tribal review process. For many years research approval was the joint responsibility of IHS and the Navajo Nation. The Navajo Nation IRB has certain core concerns that researchers are expected to address in their application, including:

- The benefits to the health of the nation and the individuals;
- Agreement that the Navajo Nation owns the collected data;
- Individualized consent forms that are thorough, exact, and truly informative for each participant, keeping in mind that a Navajo translation may be needed;
- A training component to educate local students and others about research;
- A plan for the primary investigator to report back to the tribe via IHS care providers, chapter houses, or tribal employees; and
- An agreement regarding tribal approval of manuscripts for publication and public presentations.

Researchers need to inquire about the various levels of local approval within a community. In smaller tribes, local approval may consist of a presentation to the health board, which makes a recommendation to the tribal council. Another tribe may require a presentation to an area or regional tribal entity. The Navajo Nation requires an initial approval at the chapter (small community) level, followed by resolutions of support from the IHS Health Board (if IHS will be involved in any way), the Area IHS, the Navajo Nation IRB, and the national IHS IRB. Because each tribe operates differently, the researcher needs to maintain regular communication and follow and respect policies developed by tribal nations.

## SEEKING APPROVAL EVERY STEP OF THE WAY

Many tribes are adamant that researchers first present their findings to the local health board, tribal health department, IHS providers, or the IRB prior to institutional reports. Any pertinent recommendations need to be discussed and evaluated for clarity and appropriateness. Researchers must seek prior approval with these groups before submitting publications to journals and making public presentations to peers. Tribes want to know how researchers will present their community to the world and how data will be interpreted. Another advantage of working with the tribe before publication is that it enables the researcher to discuss not only future studies but also how the current study could have been strengthened. One reason that tribes are sensitive to public presentation without tribal approval is that in a small tribe and small study sample, the researcher may inadvertently disclose the identity of study participants to other community members.

## HONORING AND INCLUDING INDIGENOUS KNOWLEDGE

Native scholars and researchers have begun to criticize the Western research epistemology of objective observation, manipulation, individuality, validity, and ownership of knowledge. By contrast, Indigenous epistemology is steeped in lessons from experiential learning, inseparability of the researcher and the subject, participant observation, interaction with nature, equality between all things in the environment, the role of elders who have lived long to acquire wisdom, a holistic perspective, connectedness, relationships, and circular learning patterns (Cajete 1999, Mihesuah and Wilson 2004, Smith 1999). Native/Indigenous authors, including Cajete, Mihesuah, Wilson, and Smith, have argued for decolonization strategies in research in efforts to reclaim Native/Indigenous history, knowledge, self-determination, cultural revitalization, and survival. Cajete (1999) speaks about Native science having different levels and meanings and laws of interdependence. Wilson (2008) writes about the value of relationships between researcher and topics as well as many elements of Native existence, including how respect, reciprocity, and responsibility are important values to uphold as Native researchers. Wilson likens research to ceremony and research as ceremony, in that research allows us to raise our level of consciousness and to build stronger relationships with our surroundings. All encourage researchers to present studies from a Native paradigm and develop Native theories and methods that could more appropriately explain challenges in Native communities.

## DEVELOPING AND IMPLEMENTING HEALTH POLICY

While most researchers would not seek to implement health policy as a result of their study with AIAN populations, the local community may request assistance in this area. As Warne (2006) indicates, the current research paradigm is a partnership between a funding agency and a research institution. Research results are defined by publications of those from the research institution and scientific findings by the funders while the community and its members serve as a laboratory or source of data (Warne 2006). Conversely, incorporating the community as equal partner would be of potential benefit to its people (current and future), as it may strengthen applications to local programs and policy development. Policy development becomes critical to protecting long-term tribal community health through programs, including strategies for local tobacco control or reducing regional or national cancer disparities (Warne 2006, Satter et al. 2012, Warne et al. 2012). Often a community poses the question, "We know we have problems with diabetes or cancer [or whatever the focus would be], but how will this study change all of that?" Policy development would require that tribal nations exercise their sovereignty to protect against increasing morbidity and mortality, as well as to provide for health promotion and cost savings. This puts the tribe or community in a proactive mode to apply research findings in the manner they prefer.

## SUMMARY

CBPR and TPR are ethical and practical, particularly when working with AIAN communities. Researchers need to be aware of the historic context of research, build trust with the community, work toward positive benefits to the community, and respect the community's culture and sovereignty. The ultimate goal of CBPR is to translate research findings into a comprehensive program that improves the health of the members of the local community while at the same time helping to develop health policy for overcoming health disparities (Tom-Orme 2002b, Warne et al. 2012).

## REFERENCES

Aaron KF, Bass EB. 2002. Community based participatory research, a call for papers. *J Gen Intern Med.* 17:84.

American Indian Law Center. 1999. *Model Tribal Research Code*. 3rd edition. Albuquerque, NM: American Indian Law Center.

Beals J, Belcourt-Dittloff A, Freedenthal S, et al. 2009. Reflections on a proposed theory of reservation-dwelling American Indian alcohol use: comment on Spillane and Smith (2007). *Psychol Bull*. 135(2):339–43; discussion 344–6.

Beauvais F. 1998. American Indians and alcohol. *Alcohol Health Res World*. 22(4):253–9.

Becker TM, Wheeler CM, McPherson RS, et al. 1993. Risk factors for cervical dysplasia in southwestern American Indian women: a pilot study. *Alaska Med*. 35(4):255–263.

Carrese JA, Rhodes LA. 1995. Western bioethics on the Navajo reservation: benefit or harm. *JAMA*. 274(10):826–829.

Cajete G. 1999. *Native Science: Natural Laws of Interdependence*. Santa Fe, NM: Clear Light Publishers.

Fisher PA, Ball TJ. 2003. Tribal participatory research: mechanisms of a collaborative model. *Am J Community Psychol*. 32(3/4):207–216.

Green LW, Mercer SL. 2001. Can public health researchers and agencies reconcile the push from funding bodies and the pull from communities? *Am J Public Health*. 91(12):1926–1942.

Hampton JW, Keala J, Luce P. 1996. Overview of national cancer institute networks for cancer control research in Native American populations. *Cancer*. 78(7):1545–1552.

Lanier AP, Kelly JJ, Holck P, et al. 2001. Cancer incidence in Alaska Natives thirty-year report 1969–1998. *Alaska Med*. 43(4):87–115.

Leininger M. 1970. *Nursing and Anthropology: Two Worlds to Blend*. New York, NY: John Wiley.

Leininger M, McFarland MR. 2002. *Transcultural Nursing: Concepts, Theories, Research, and Practice*. 3rd edition. New York, NY: McGraw-Hill Companies Inc.

Mihesuah DA, Wilson AC. 2004. *Indigenizing the Academy: Transforming Scholarship and Empowering Communities*. Lincoln, NE: University of Nebraska Press.

Petereit DG, Burhansstipanov L. 2008. Establishing trusting partnerships for successful recruitment of American Indians to clinical trials. *Cancer Control*. 15(3):260–268.

Petereit DG, Molloy K, Reiner ML, et al. 2008. Establishing a patient navigator program to reduce cancer disparities in the American Indian communities of western South Dakota: initial observations and results. *Cancer Control.* 15(3):254–259.

Potvin L, Cargo M, McComber AM, et al. 2003. Implementing participatory intervention and research in communities: lessons from the Kahnawake schools diabetes prevention project in Canada. *Soc Sci Med.* 56(6):1295–1305.

Satter DE, Roby DH, Smith LM, et al. 2012. Costs of smoking and policy strategies for California American Indian communities. *J Cancer Educ.* 27(supp 1):S91–105.

Smith LT. 1999. *Decolonizing Methodologies: Research and Indigenous Peoples.* New York, NY: Zed Books.

Strickland CJ. 1999. Conducting focus groups cross-culturally: experiences with Pacific Northwest Indian People. *Public Health Nurs.* 16(3):190–197.

Tom-Orme L. 1991. The search for insider-outsider partnerships in research. In: Hibbard H, Nutting PA, Grady ML, editors. *AHCPR Conference Proceedings: Primary Care Research: Theory and Methods.* Washington, DC: Agency for Health Care Policy and Research, Department of Health and Human Services. p. 229–233.

Tom-Orme L. 2000. Native Americans explaining illness: storytelling as illness experience. In: Whaley BB, editor. *Explaining Illness: Research, Theory, and Strategies.* Mahwah, NJ: Lawrence Erlbaum Associates. p. 237–257.

Tom-Orme L. 2002a. Opinion: what are the ethical concerns that must be addressed when conducting medical research with people of different cultures? *Health Sciences Report.* Salt Lake City: University of Utah. Available at: http://healthcare.utah.edu/publicaffairs/publications/HSR/Archive/summer2002/opinion.html. Accessed September 11, 2013.

Tom-Orme L. 2002b. Transcultural nursing and health care among Native Americans. In: Leininger M, McFarland MR, editors. *Transcultural Nursing: Concepts, Theories, Research, and Practice.* New York, NY: McGraw Hill Medical Publishing Division. p. 429–440.

Wallerstein NB, Duran B. 2006. Using community-based participatory research to address health disparities. *Health Promot Pract.* 3:312–23.

Warne D. 2006. Research and educational approaches to reducing health disparities among American Indians and Alaska Natives. *J Transcultural Nurs.* 17(3):266–271.

Warne D, Kaur J, Perdue D. 2012. American Indian/Alaska Native cancer policy: systemic approaches to reducing cancer disparities. *J Canc Educ.* 27(Suppl 1):S18–S23.

Wilson S. 2008. *Research is Ceremony: Indigenous Research Methods.* Halifax, Nova Scotia: Fernwood Publishing.

# 8

# Examples of Successful Community-Based Participatory Research in American Indian Communities

Thomas K. Welty, MD, MPH

## INTRODUCTION

While all federally funded biomedical research in the United States requires review and approval by an institutional review board (IRB) or ethics committee, few researchers take into consideration the concerns of the community in which they are conducting their studies. Research conducted in academic healthcare facilities usually does not require review and approval by city or state governments. Thus, many capable researchers are not familiar with the concept of participatory research at the community level that has become the standard of research in American Indian (AI) communities.

Often there is an unfounded fear on the part of researchers that submission of research proposals for community or tribal review and approval will necessitate changes in the protocol that will compromise the quality of the research. Similarly, there is concern that submission of scientific manuscripts for community or tribal review and approval prior to publication will result in restriction of free speech. Also, it is worth noting that the time and costs involved in obtaining community/tribal review and approvals are substantial.

More emphasis is needed in academic environments on the importance of community-based participatory research as a means of increasing the benefits of the research to those communities. Researchers must learn how to explain complex scientific proposals in terms that lay people can understand. Learning this skill will increase the value of research to the entire community, not just to a small group of academic researchers who often do not carefully consider how their research can benefit the communities they are studying. At the same time, community leaders need to learn as much as possible about common health problems in their communities and recruit capable researchers to study those problems in a way that produces maximal health benefit for the community/ tribe and the study participants. When they receive unsolicited research proposals, they should review them carefully and make constructive, culturally appropriate suggestions that will enhance the benefits to the communities. Usually, such changes do not compromise the scientific value of the study. The goal is for the community/tribal leaders and researchers to have a collegial relationship that has the greatest likelihood of creating new knowledge that results in improved health for American Indians. Several studies of Indian health problems that have achieved this goal are described below.

## CARDIOVASCULAR DISEASE

In 1988, the National Heart, Lung and Blood Institute (NHLBI) of the National Institutes of Health released a Request for Application for a cooperative agreement study of cardiovascular disease (CVD) and its risk factors among American Indians. Because some scientists raised questions on whether the recruitment goals of 1,500 participants aged 45 to 74 years in each of three sites could be achieved, all applicants had to demonstrate expertise in working with tribal communities. Each of the awardees (University of Oklahoma, Medlantic Research Institute, and the Aberdeen Area Indian Health Service Epidemiology Program) had successfully conducted previous research in Indian communities and had good working relationships with those communities (Lee et al. 1990, Stoddart et al. 2000, Sambo 2001). The participating tribes provided input into the study design and implementation, including suggesting the name Strong Heart Study (SHS). This input enabled the study to attain its recruitment goals.

The investigators made frequent presentations of the results to the tribal communities and obtained approval to conduct two follow-up examinations on all of the participants. The study was designed to maximize the benefits to the tribal communities and participants. The SHS participants received three thorough medical examinations, including lipid profiles, glucose tolerance tests, echocardiograms, electrocardiograms, tuberculin tests, pulmonary function tests, and carotid ultrasound tests. Clinically useful information was shared with their providers and, occasionally, critical medical conditions were detected that required immediate follow up. In addition, all participants were given educational brochures and advice on how they could improve their health by undergoing Indian-specific health risk appraisals (Welty 1988, Welty et al. 1989). In the Dakota Center, the National Cancer Institute (NCI) funded an ancillary study called the Sioux Cancer Study, which enabled researchers to screen all female participants for cervical cancer by Pap smears and pelvic examination, for breast cancer by clinical breast exams and mammograms, and for rectal cancer by rectal examinations and occult blood testing (Welty et al. 1993). All male participants were screened for prostate and rectal cancer by rectal examinations and occult blood testing. Through this screening of 1532 Dakota Center SHS participants, four cancers were diagnosed and participants were referred for definitive surgical procedures earlier than they would have been if they had not participated in the SHS. The Sioux Cancer Study also raised the awareness of cancer screening in the Dakota Center communities.

The participating tribal communities benefited by gaining experience in conducting research. A total of 139 community members, including many students in health professions, worked on the SHS during the first three phases. Many AI students decided to pursue higher education goals as a result of their involvement in the SHS and subsequently returned to their communities to pursue research or to provide healthcare (Sambo 2001).

Since the National Health and Nutrition Examination Surveys, Health Interview Surveys, and Behavioral Risk Factor Surveys do not usually include enough American Indians to estimate the prevalence of health problems and risk factors, the SHS data have been cited as the best estimate of health problems and risk factors among American Indians. However, the SHS was not designed to be a representative sample of American Indians, and the study results clearly demonstrate regional and tribal differences in health problems and CVD risk. While the aggregate data may appropriately describe AI health problems at the national level, regional or tribe-specific data are more appropriate to design and implement community-based interventions for prevention of health problems, so they can be tailored to address different risk factors in each community (Welty 1995).

The SHS also provided a unique opportunity to study other chronic illnesses in American Indians. With appropriate IRB and tribal approvals, much has been learned about sleep disorders, asthma, and other pulmonary diseases (Marion et al. 2001, Quan et al. 1997, National Heart Lung and Blood Institute 2012). In 2002, the NCI funded a multicenter longitudinal study of chronic diseases in American Indians and Alaska Natives, which was called the EARTH (Education and Research Toward Health) Study. The SHS staff shared their protocols and expertise with the EARTH Study investigators to help them plan and implement their research (Slattery et al. 2007).

The third examination of the SHS cohort included a pilot family study to investigate genetic factors associated with CVD. The tribal communities requested that SHS investigators include younger participants in the study, which was done in phase three as part of the family study. The investigators reassured the community that this genetic study would be done according to tribal values and wishes. The SHS staff did not clone cells because the tribes did not want this procedure done. Instead, other techniques were used so that the study was still scientifically valid. Because of the collaborative working relationships that SHS investigators had with the participating tribal communities, the pilot study was successful in recruiting 900 family members of the original cohort to participate. The fourth phase of the SHS expanded the number of family members to 2700, so that the study had sufficient power to perform genetic mapping for CVD risk factors (North et al. 2003). SHS investigators have completed a fifth phase of the study to further investigate genetic factors associated with CVD. In 2013, NHLBI funded a sixth phase of the study for five years, which will support continued surveillance of morbidity and mortality among original participants and family study participants. A complete listing of all SHS publications as well as questionnaires and standard operating procedures for all phases can be found at http://strongheart.ouhsc.edu.

While the Framingham Study of Cardiovascular Disease has provided important general knowledge about CVD, the SHS has provided more specific knowledge about CVD in American Indians, and much of that knowledge is also applicable to all humankind. The SHS also has confirmed the role of obesity as the major preventable risk factor that causes the epidemic of diabetes and the subsequent CVD currently afflicting American Indians. As a result, NHLBI subsequently funded the Pathways Study to investigate interventions for the primary prevention of obesity in AI children (Gittelsohn et al. 2003). SHS researchers also submitted a proposal to NHBLI to prevent atherosclerosis in AI persons with diabetes. The SANDS Study (Stop Atherosclerosis in Native Diabetics Study), a multicenter clinical trial funded in 2002, found that aggressive treatment of hypertension and hyperlipidemia among American Indians with diabetes resulted in a decrease in carotid atherosclerosis as determined by ultrasound measurement of intimal medial common cartotid artery thickness, whereas those participants who received standard treatment had an increase in intimal medial thickness (Howard et al. 2008). These findings have led to improved clinical care for AI patients with diabetes. Continuing input from tribal people is essential for SHS investigators to use their expertise to fully realize the potential that cardiovascular disease research has for improving the health of tribal communities. The highest priority is to develop effective clinical and community-based interventions that will reduce the incidence and prevalence of obesity and its sequelae (diabetes, CVD, and other related chronic diseases).

## OTHER GENETIC STUDIES

While there are many cultural considerations in doing genetic research among American Indians, the key to success is community involvement with the researchers, which can lead to clinical and public health benefits for the participants and communities. For example, genetic research that began in the 1980s identified a cancer gene that increased the risk of nonpolyposis colon cancer among a Navajo family with high morbidity and mortality rates from colon cancer. The results of this research led to individual genetic counseling for the entire family that tailored colon cancer screening based on the results of genetic testing (Lynch et al. 1996).

Another example of mutually successful genetic research was undertaken with the Zuni Tribe, which has a very high rate of renal disease, much of it related to IgA nephropathy. Genetic studies done by researchers, who had long-term relationships with the tribe, found that much of the renal disease within the community is related to genetic factors. Those researchers continue to work with the tribe to promote appropriate interventions (MacCluer et al. 2010).

## MATERNAL AND CHILD HEALTH

### Sudden Infant Death Syndrome

Indian families treasure their children and experience great pain and suffering when they die suddenly and unexpectedly. For that reason, Northern Plains tribal leaders and communities were anxious to use all available tools of Western medicine in the 1990s to investigate why so many Indian babies were dying of sudden infant death syndrome (SIDS). A team of researchers from the Centers for Disease Control and Prevention (CDC), the National Institute of Child Health and Development, the Indian Health Service (IHS), and various academic institutions developed a protocol to investigate such deaths, including autopsies and neuropathologic studies (Randall and Randall 1999).

After consultation with spiritual leaders on the appropriateness of conducting such investigations and incorporating their suggestions, the investigators developed a protocol that was reviewed and approved by nine tribes as well as multiple IRBs, tribal organizations, and the Medicine Wheel Coalition of medicine men from states near the Black Hills of South Dakota, (Randall et al. 2001). This process took over a year and resulted in improvements in the protocol from scientific and cultural perspectives (Gittelsohn et al. 2003). Parents of children who died in the first year of life and parents of children who lived were interviewed by AI nurses. Only a small number of parents refused to participate in the study (Randall et al. 2001). Throughout this five-year study and the subsequent five years it took to analyze and publish the results, the investigators kept the tribal communities and leaders informed of the study's progress and its results. Public health nurse visits were found to be helpful in preventing SIDS, while maternal alcohol abuse and overbundling the baby with blankets were found to be risk factors (Iyasu et al. 2002). Similar results for maternal alcohol use were found in a recent study by O'Leary et al. (2013). The tribal leaders encouraged the investigators to publish the results in a widely circulated journal, so that this knowledge could benefit as many people as possible and lead to preventive interventions that would result in a reduction of SIDS. They are committed to doing all they can to reduce the rates of SIDS in their communities. This study would not have been possible to complete without the ongoing partnership between the scientific community and the tribal community, which began before the study started and continued throughout the data collection and analytic phases. Reducing SIDS rates for Northern Plains Indians will require ongoing collaboration among tribal leaders and communities, healthcare providers, and researchers. Other studies have been generated from this research to increase knowledge related to SIDS and its risk factors. Health education material specific to Native communities has been developed. This material utilizes the knowledge gained from these studies, such as Native Generations from the Urban Indian Health Institute (http://www.uihi.org) and Healthy Native Babies (https://www.nichd.nih.gov/publications/Pages/pubs_details.aspx?pubs_id=5733).

## *Maternal Substance Use*

Tribal leaders recognize the damage that maternal alcohol abuse causes to unborn children and are anxious to reduce or eliminate fetal alcohol spectrum disorders (FASD) and other alcohol-related developmental disabilities (ARDD) from their communities. In 1993, the Aberdeen Area Tribal Chairmen's Health Board received a grant to reduce ARDD in their communities by establishing volunteer community response teams to develop prevention plans in each of the 19 tribal communities. As part of this effort, they supported a study to validate a screening tool for maternal substance use and to study women who had children with FASD or some characteristics of FASD (formerly called fetal alcohol syndrome [FAS] or fetal alcohol exposure or effects [FAE]). Subsequently, the researchers validated the screening tool, which is now available on the IHS Web site for use by prenatal care providers (Bull et al. 1999). Women who have a child with FASD or some characteristics of FASD have many medical and social needs that healthcare providers should address so these women can regain their self-esteem and stop using alcohol during future pregnancies to prevent FASD (Kvigne et al. 2003). Follow-up investigations of mothers who had a child with FASD have shown that children born after a child with FASD was born had better outcomes, a finding that was associated with a decrease in maternal alcohol consumption during the after-sibling pregnancy (Kvigne et al. 2009).

In order to reduce FASD and ARDD in Indian communities, tribal leaders, IHS, and researchers need to collaborate in the training of healthcare providers regarding how to screen for substance use in pregnant patients and how to intervene to reduce or eliminate fetal alcohol exposure. More research is needed to determine the most effective intervention for women of childbearing age who are abusing alcohol, including how to motivate fathers to be helpful in promoting abstinence during pregnancy.

## INFECTIOUS DISEASE

### Vaccine Development

Historically, AI communities have been plagued by high rates of infectious diseases, and for that reason many researchers have conducted vaccine trials in those communities. Communities that have high rates of diseases will benefit the most if the vaccine works. Fewer study participants from such communities are needed to confirm the efficacy of the vaccine because the incidence of disease is high. In addition, the efficacy of some vaccines varies among populations, so conducting vaccine research in Indian communities more definitively establishes how well the vaccine will work in AI populations.

Hepatitis A is an example of an infectious disease that has plagued AI communities. During the 1970s and 1980s, hepatitis A occurred in community-wide epidemics in Northern Plains Indian communities every five to seven years, resulting in a seroprevalence of hepatitis A IgG antibodies of 90% in persons aged 20 years and older (Shaw et al. 1990). In 1993, investigators from IHS and CDC obtained IRB and tribal/community approvals to conduct an immunogenicity trial of an experimental hepatitis A vaccine in infants and an efficacy trial in children aged 5 to 12 years. Tribal support for the efficacy trial was withdrawn because of concerns regarding the safety of the vaccine, although their concerns were not substantiated. Subsequently, the immunogenic response trial in infants was completed with the ongoing support of the tribal community, and demonstrated that the immunogenic response to the vaccine was reduced in children who had maternal antibodies to hepatitis A (Letson et al. 2004). For that reason, the vaccine was licensed for use in children older than two years, when maternal antibodies had waned. Further research on its use in children younger than two years continues.

After licensure, the hepatitis A vaccine was widely administered to AI children over two years of age, and the periodic epidemics of hepatitis A in those communities have stopped. Thus, this research was extremely beneficial to Indian communities, as it led to a licensure of a vaccine that greatly reduced a serious infectious disease in children from those communities. In retrospect, more intensive dialogue between the investigators and communities prior to initiating the efficacy study may have enabled it to be completed as well.

Similarly in this same time period, pneumococcal disease rates were much higher in some AI communities than in other populations. A conjugate pneumococcal vaccine trial was conducted among southwestern AI infants, and the vaccine subsequently was found to be immunogenic (Moulton et al. 2001, Miernyk et al. 2000). This vaccine is now licensed and has the potential to reduce rates of pneumonia, otitis media, septicemia, and meningitis in American Indians. Immunizations remain an important component of Indian healthcare, and research in Indian communities continues to contribute greatly to the development and use of efficacious vaccines (Committee on Native American Child Health and Committee on Infectious Diseases 1999).

## Tuberculosis

Historically, tuberculosis (TB) has been a serious health problem for American Indians (Rieder 1989). Through prompt treatment of cases, contact tracing, and treatment of latent TB, incidence rates have decreased but are still much higher than in other populations. Navajo tribal involvement in TB control, through the efforts of councilwoman Annie Wauneka and others, led to the development in 1972 of the tribe-run Navajo Tribal TB Control Program. Previously, some of the clinical trials on the efficacy of isoniazid (INH), one of the major drugs for treating TB, were conducted on the Navajo reservation.

As a result of improved control, transmission of TB in Indian communities has decreased greatly, and few children and young adults are now infected by *Mycobacterium tuberculosis*. However, the rates of latent TB infection remain as high as 70% in older persons in some Indian communities, and those high rates of latent disease cause the persistently high incidence rates of active TB (Breault and Hoffman 1997).

Research among Oglala Sioux Indians demonstrates that persons with diabetes have a five-fold increased risk of latent TB progressing to active TB; however, studies have also found that chemoprophylaxis in persons with latent

TB reduces the risk of the development of active TB. Further investigation has indicated that treatment of diabetic patients who have latent TB with INH could prevent 55% of TB cases in that tribe (Breault and Hoffman 1997). While HIV infection is a risk factor for TB among American Indians, the epidemic of diabetes in this population has contributed more to the high rates of TB than have HIV infections. The IHS Diabetes Control Program has included screening for TB and treatment of latent disease as part of their quality of care monitor (Giroux and Skipper 2003). This research has led to improvements in care that will accelerate the decline in TB incidence among American Indians.

## SUMMARY

This chapter provides several examples of research that have contributed to improvements in the health of American Indians. These examples demonstrate that the investigators worked with the tribal communities in a collaborative manner, and that this partnership was responsible for the success of the research.

## ACKNOWLEDGMENTS

The Aberdeen Area Tribal Chairmen's Health Board and the tribal leaders and communities in the Aberdeen Area provided input and support that enabled the research described in this report to succeed. The IRBs provided useful input into the study design and implementation. The investigators had the patience and perseverance to successfully collaborate with the tribal communities. The opinions expressed in this report are those of the author and are not necessarily those of the Indian Health Service.

## REFERENCES

Breault JL, Hoffman MG. 1997. A strategy for reducing tuberculosis among Oglala Sioux Native Americans. *Am J Prev Med.* 13(3):182–188.

Bull LB, Kvigne VL, Leonardson GR, et al. 1999. Validation of a self-administered questionnaire to screen for prenatal alcohol use in Northern Plains Indian women. *Am J Prev Med.* 16(3):240–3.

Committee on Native American Child Health and Committee on Infectious Diseases, American Academy of Pediatrics. 1999. Immunizations for Native American children. *Pediatrics.* 104(3 Pt 1):564–567.

Giroux JA, Skipper B. 2003. *Preventing Tuberculosis in American Indian and Alaska Native Who Have Diabetes: Can We Do More?* [Master's thesis.] Minneapolis, MN: University of Minnesota.

Gittelsohn J, Davis SM, Steckler A, et al. 2003. Pathways: lessons learned and future directions for school-based interventions among American Indians. *Prev Med.* 37(6 Pt 2):S107–12.

Howard BV, Roman MJ, Devereux RB, et al. 2008. Effect of lower targets for blood pressure and LDL cholesterol on atherosclerosis in diabetes: the SANDS randomized trial. *JAMA.* 299(14):1678–89.

Iyasu S, Randall LL, Welty TK, et al. 2002. Risk factors for Sudden Infant Death Syndrome among Northern Plains Indians. *JAMA.* 288:2717–2723.

Kvigne VL, Leonardson GR, Borzelleca J, et al. 2003. Characteristics of mothers who have children with fetal alcohol syndrome or some characteristics of fetal alcohol syndrome. *J Am Board Fam Pract.* 16(4):296–303.

Kvigne VL, Leonardson GR, Borzelleca J, et al. 2009. Characteristics of children whose siblings have fetal alcohol syndrome or incomplete fetal alcohol syndrome. *Pediatrics.* 123(3):e526–33.

Lee ET, Welty TK, Fabsitz R, et al. 1990. The Strong Heart Study. A study of cardiovascular disease in American Indians: design and methods. *Am J Epidemiol.* 132(6):1141–55.

Letson GW, Shapiro CN, Kuehn D, et al. 2004. Effect of maternal antibody on immunogenicity of hepatitis A vaccine in infants. *J Pediatr.* 144(3):327–32.

Lynch HT, Drouhard T, Vasen HF, et al. 1996. Genetic counseling in a Navajo hereditary nonpolyposis colorectal cancer kindred. *Cancer.* 77(1):30–5.

MacCluer JW, Scavini M, Shah VO, et al. 2010. Heritability of measures of kidney disease among Zuni Indians: The Zuni Kidney Project. *Am J Kidney Dis.* 56:289–302.

Marion MS, Leonardson GR, Rhoades ER, et al. 2001. Spirometry reference values for American Indian adults: results from the Strong Heart Study. *Chest.* 120(2):489–95.

Miernyk KM, Parkinson AJ, Rudolph KM, et al. 2000. Immunogenicity of a heptavalent pneumococcal conjugate vaccine in Apache and Navajo Indian, Alaska native, and non-native American children aged <2 years. *Clin Infect Dis.* 31(1):34–41.

Moulton LH, O'Brien KL, Kohberger R, et al. 2001. Design of a group-randomized Streptococcus pneumoniae vaccine trial. *Control Clin Trials*22(4):438–52.

National Heart Lung and Blood Institute, National Institutes of Health. *The Sleep Heart Health Study: Bibliography.* Available at: http://www.jhucct.com/shhs/details/biblio.htm. Accessed February 23, 2013.

North KE, Howard BV, Welty TK, et al. 2003. Genetic and environmental contributions to cardiovascular disease risk in American Indians: the strong heart family study. *Am J Epidemiol.* 157(4):303–14.

O'Leary CM, Jacoby PJ, Bartu A, et al. 2013. Maternal alcohol use and sudden infant death syndrome and infant mortality excluding SIDS. *Pediatrics.* February 25, 2013 [Epub ahead of print].

Quan SF, Howard BV, Iber C, et al. 1997. The Sleep Heart Health Study: design, rationale, and methods. *Sleep.* 20(12):1077–85.

Randall LL, Krogh C, Welty TK, et al. 2001. The Aberdeen Indian Health Service Infant Mortality Study: design, methodology and implementation. *Am Indian Alsk Native Ment Health Res.* 10(1):1–20.

Randall B, Randall LL. 1999. Initiation of formal death investigation procedures amongst the Northern Plains Indians: a necessary adjunct in the study of American Indian sudden infant deaths. *Am J Forensic Med Pathol.* 20(1):22–6.

Rieder HL. 1989. Tuberculosis among American Indians of the contiguous United States. *Public Health Rep.* 104(6):653–7.

Sambo BH; Strong Heart Study Investigators. 2001. The Strong Heart Study: interaction with and benefit to American Indian communities. *Am J Med Sci.* 322(5):282–5.

Shaw FE Jr, Shapiro CN, Welty TK, et al. 1990. Hepatitis transmission among the Sioux Indians of South Dakota. *Am J Public Health.* 80(9):1091–4.

Slattery ML, Schumacher MC, Lanier AP, et al. 2007. A prospective cohort of American Indian and Alaska Native people: study design, methods, and implementation. *Am J Epidemiol.* 166(5):606–15.

Stoddart ML, Jarvis B, Blake B, et al. 2000. Recruitment of American Indians in epidemiologic research: The Strong Heart Study. *Am Indian Alsk Native Ment Health Res.* 9(3):20–37.

Welty TK. 1988. Indian specific health risk appraisal developed. *IHS Primary Care Provider.* 13:65.

Welty TK. 1989. Finding the Way—Indian Specific HRA Released. *IHS Primary Care Provider.* 13:64–65.

Welty TK, Lee E, Yeh JL, et al. 1995. Cardiovascular disease risk factors among American Indians. The Strong Heart Study. *Am J Epidemiology.*, 1995, 142:264–287.

Welty TK, Zephier N, Schweigman K, et al. 1993. Cancer risk factors in three Sioux tribes. Use of the Indian-specific health risk appraisal for data collection and analysis. *Alaska Med.* 35(4):265–72.

# 9

# Case Studies: Projects Gone Awry

Teshia G. Arambula Solomon, PhD

## INTRODUCTION

Four published case studies in the Native American (NA) community that had negative interactions will be examined in this chapter, and options and actions that may have prevented misunderstandings and could have improved the outcomes will be explored (Wallerstein 1999, Shah 2000, Swenson 2001, Associated Press 2001, Foulks 1989, Bommersbach 2008, NY Times 2010). We will discuss what went wrong in each study, despite any good intentions the investigators may have had.

## CASE ONE: FIVE MILES FROM TOMORROW

In October 2000, the *Journal of the American Medical Association* (*JAMA*) published a letter by a young medical student, Shetal Shah, telling of the suicide of an elderly Alaska Native. Shah describes the village he worked in during his rotation as "an Arctic afterthought of a human settlement." After naming the tribal community, he adds: "Although this is US territory, English is rarely spoken outside the three-room schoolhouse, and diversity means not sharing one of three common surnames on the island." He also refers to the village as one that "has fallen off the map" (2000).

In the letter, Shah relates a tale of a 97-year-old great whale hunter who presented in the clinic with a case of what the patient called "uselessness." His end-of-life experience included the patient, attending physician, and the patient's family gathered in prayer to celebrate the elder's decision. Shah discusses the medical ethics of condoning such action, particularly without an obvious illness in the patient. He ends his tale by recounting the Native elder's last day as he stepped onto an icecap and "smiles toothlessly, waves, and slowly vanishes into the early morning fog."

In August of the following year, *JAMA* printed a rebuttal to Shah's letter by Dr. Michael D. Swenson, the attending physician supervising his work. Swenson commends Shah for raising the question of end-of-life ethics but notes that Shah's article was presented as a true story when in fact it was not. Swenson adds that in the community in which he works, there is no tribal tradition whereby an elder bids farewell to his family and walks into the ocean. He explains the custom of valuing elders and adds that the story reinforces cultural prejudices. Swenson also remarks that suicide might be a more appropriate response to uselessness in a (Western) culture in which status is dependent upon performance and achievements, than in a Native culture, which has a different value system (2001).

In his rebuttal Shah states that he had taken literary license by creating a compilation of stories told to him in his five-week stay in Alaska and that "the ultimate purpose of the story was hopefully served, and the medical community can concentrate more on end-of-life issues and less on stylized writing." He stood by his account, saying:

> Being held in high regard [as an elder] by peers does not necessarily translate to feeling useful in a part of the world where living is extremely difficult. Such feelings have, I believe, led several older members of the [tribe] to take the actions I discussed.

At the bottom of Shah's letter is an editor's note stating that *JAMA* had believed the manuscript related an actual experience. On August 21, 2001, the Associated Press published an article stating that *JAMA* was "duped" by the story. Although the article focused on *JAMA* being misled, the author listed the tribe and community by name.

No one would consider a tourist to be an expert in a culture. Five weeks in any community is not long enough to understand a people, their history, or their traditions. Shah not only took literary license, but also cultural license. He broke confidentiality by disclosing the geographic location and the tribal name of the community. In small communities it is easy to determine who is being spoken about when specific details are disclosed. Shah was disrespectful in his description of the community as an "afterthought." Rich traditions exist in remote communities, and the peoples of those communities often choose to live in their homelands despite the hardships of doing so. The letter written by Shah and published by *JAMA* disregarded both professional and research ethics.

When working in Native communities, permission must be obtained from the tribal committee that oversees the protection of human participants, such as the institutional review board (IRB). These committees also exercise some oversight on dissemination of the data and whether reports may contain the name of the tribe or the community being studied. Seemingly innocent information, such as geographic location, can easily break confidentiality and identify the community, an ethical breech that abuses privacy rights. By working with the IRB, authors can avoid disclosing confidential and potentially harmful information.

Medical and other health professional interns are guests in these communities. Medical schools and other academic institutions should establish and advise students about IRB protocols and professional ethics. Scientific journals, as with other forms of journalism, also have a responsibility to check the accuracy of articles and provide disclaimers when appropriate.

## CASE TWO: HEALTHIER COMMUNITIES

In her article, "Power Between Evaluator and Community" Wallerstein (1999) describes the power struggle between a researcher and communities she observed while serving as an evaluator for the Healthier Communities (HC) initiative in New Mexico. The HC project, based on a partnership that included private and public agencies, individuals, schools, universities, and tribal communities, was launched in 1992 to improve the quality of life for children and families. Wallerstein was hired to provide an international perspective and create the overall framework for the project. Funding was allocated to a nonprofit agency by the state through community bidding. The nonprofit agency was to be an intermediary between the state department of health and local communities.

During the second year of the project, a number of problems arose. A new agency became the intermediary, and this agency had neither a clear commitment to communities nor a mission of prevention. New leadership in the state office left the project with limited resources and a lack of direction. Community leaders expressed conflicting ideas about the vision of healthier communities and had difficulties in translating an abstract set of principles into concrete action. Furthermore, three out of four of the project coordinators rejected the expectation that their coalitions should be judged on the stated project principles. Tension increased between the communities and the state agencies, offices, and representatives. The communities were unhappy with state purchasing and reimbursement procedures and the lack of an effective process for managing grants and contracts. There was a lack of communication between community and state personnel and even among and within state agencies. The communities became skeptical about the state's sincerity in shared community decision-making and felt that the state did not respect the communities' sovereignty. Thus, power struggles permeated the project: within communities, between agency departments, and between the state agencies and the communities. Power imbalances were reflected when some individuals were left out of the communication loop and had little or no decision-making authority.

In this power struggle, the communities viewed Wallerstein as part of the state government and the power structure. Community members believed that the evaluation would influence future funding decisions and that she had the power to control how the state would direct the work. Coalition coordinators felt that they could not refuse to participate in the evaluation, despite viewing the process as a nuisance rather than as a useful planning tool. Their resistance was expressed by controlling who would be interviewed. As a result, the evaluation plan was ultimately not sufficient to gain coordinator support, build trust, or develop a community agenda.

The project findings, which acknowledged areas of conflict between the research team and the communities, were rejected by the communities and coalition board members, who demonstrated their disappointment by boycotting feedback sessions. In three communities where a lack of diversity and representation of minority constituencies in the coalition had been cited, coalition members were defensive, citing "outsider" interpretation, and the evaluation report was ultimately ignored. Wallerstein states that she circumvented community resistance to the evaluation by interviewing people referred to her by other community members and by not clearing the referrals with the project coordinators who developed the list of participants to be interviewed. She justified her actions as a scientific decision, and did not confront the political problems that had arisen between the communities and the state agencies.

In addition, meetings were held in the state capital, forcing community coordinators to travel to the state capital to meet with Wallerstein instead of her traveling to their communities. Commenting on this power imbalance, one outreach worker observed: "People in the capital believe it is a longer drive from Albuquerque to [here], than from [here] to Albuquerque."

In her analysis, Wallerstein suggests that she should have discussed the "power dynamics" up front in order to avoid the mistrust she encountered. Had community participants understood her role and had she understood their concerns, the results could have been more productive. For example, she could have hired workers from the community instead of graduate students from the university. Also, using the community's definitions of success instead of those of the World Health Organization would have illustrated true community participation. Finally, this example illustrates the importance of maintaining a regular presence in the field when conducting research in Native communities, if not in person then via phone or through other means of communication.

## CASE THREE: ALASKA ALCOHOL PROJECT

Foulks (1989), in his examination of the political and ethical dilemmas encountered in an alcohol study in Alaska, describes a classic example of unintended negative effects of research on Native communities. In this study, researchers were contracted to examine the causes of alcohol abuse in a specific village and to evaluate that village's detoxification detention program. Eighty-eight Natives were interviewed about their alcohol use and drinking behavior. Data were reported based on acculturation categories of traditional and nontraditional Natives, participation in church membership, and economic influences. The results indicated high rates of self-reported excessive drinking and pointed to the negative social consequences of alcohol consumption.

A technical advisory group of health professionals (primarily non-Native) as well as a steering committee of Native leaders helped develop and implement the project and reviewed the study results. The Native elders found the report useful as a call for change in the community. However, non-Natives in the technical advisory group felt the report had imposed inappropriate "Western, lower-48 standards on the [Native] society." They pointed out that non-Natives were not included in the study and that mentioning ancestry would be problematic. Therefore, they decided to hold a public meeting to discuss the findings of the study and to receive feedback from the community. The Native elders on the steering committee approved of the town meeting idea and the local media was used to publicize the meeting. The invitation allowed citizens to call in with questions. In addition, the research team decided to publish two reports: (1) a summary report of the results with policy recommendations, and (2) an official report that was more technical and scientific in nature that focused on the effects of social change.

Unknown to the research team, a non-Native faculty member from the local university obtained a copy of the summary report given to him by a Native friend. In a stinging letter to the local newspaper, he publicly questioned the methodology and described the study as another form of "cultural imperialism." His message was accompanied by a letter signed by individuals from the agency that funded the study, rescinding their participation in the project. Despite this development, the area's department of public safety and the contracted research agency, along with the director of public health, proceeded with the town meeting and sent out press releases reporting that the study found 50% of the adult population suffered from alcohol problems. This action was a strategy to "shock" the Native community into action.

Prior to the town meeting the research team, without consulting the community, released to the press the results previously presented to the village advisory group and steering committee. The press release resulted in a *New York Times* story headlined, "Alcohol Plagues Eskimos." An Associated Press story reported that alcoholism and violence had consumed Eskimo society as a result of newly established oil production and a United Press International Wire Service story headlined, "Sudden Wealth Sparks Epidemic of Alcoholism: What We Have Here is a Society of Alcoholics" (Foulks 1989). In addition, the borough public information officer released a report stating that the "community was stunned and angered by the content of the study, and that the manner of its release had done irreparable harm to the community" (Foulks 1989). The borough then fired the director of public safety.

In recounting this experience, Foulks states, "The press confirmed the stereotype of the drunken [Native], whose traditional culture had been plundered. The public exposure had brought shame on the community, and the people were now angry and defensive." The public meeting attracted 300 Natives, who stayed for discussion into the early hours of the morning. The researchers presented their findings and answered questions from the community members, both in English and in the Native language. In the end, the research was met with further criticism when the funding agency recruited another institution to evaluate the study. These evaluators questioned the statistical methods utilized in the study and recommended caution in accepting the recommendations. Subsequently, when presenting a paper on the research at an international health symposium, the agency health director publicly discounted the work.

Foulks notes that the project was funded and supported by only a few of the community members and therefore did not reflect the needs and attitudes of the larger community. These individuals allowed the scientific reports to become public relations tools for the mass media. He recommends that in future studies, policies and procedures be jointly developed by the research team and the community. He notes that, in general, research is first published in scientific journals prior to other media and is therefore protected by the peer review process, which lends credibility to the work. Foulks adds that "Scientists must self-consciously include these sometimes intangible, value-laden factors into their research design and planning."

## CASE FOUR: HAVASUPAI VERSUS ARIZONA BOARD OF REGENTS

One of the most egregious cases of research misconduct in Native communities is what has come to be known as the Havasupai case. In March 2004 the Havasupai, the tribe whose reservation is at the bottom of the Grand Canyon, filed a lawsuit against the Arizona Board of Regents (ABOR), charging that research was conducted without consent of the individuals and the community (Bommersbach 2008). This case is well published and the Bommersbach article in *Phoenix Magazine* (2008) does an excellent job of describing the details. Highlights of the case follow.

Essentially, what started out as good intentions on the part of tribal members and a researcher to search for a genetic link to diabetes became the example of why Native people are so distrustful of research. The research failed to comprehend the culture of the community and, according to published accounts, failed to follow human participant protection protocols and basic research ethics (Bommersbach 2008).

The Havasupai understood that participants would provide blood samples for genetic testing for diabetes, and that the blood samples would be kept at Arizona State University. However, the investigative report performed on behalf of the university (Bommersbach 2008) provides evidence that the principal investigator did not provide adequate consent to participants that their blood would be used for research purposes other than diabetes-related ones or that they could be used by other researchers without further consent from the community or the individuals. The blood samples were then used to study schizophrenia and inbreeding and unauthorized hand prints were used to study migration theories, all subject matter that most tribes would find offensive and would not approve. The specimens were also sent to other universities for analysis, something the tribe did not approve. The report suggests that:

- Blood samples were drawn prior to IRB approval;
- Schizophrenia was the primary study and no genetic diabetes research was undertaken;
- Subsequent studies by students and other investigators did not go through IRB processes and did not seek tribal consent; and
- Consent forms were either only collected in the first year of a four-year study or at least were not secure and were "lost."

The case was settled on April 20, 2010, after seven years of litigation and attempts at reconciliation. But during the litigation process, the tribe banished researchers from the reservation and other tribes in Arizona followed suit. Since this case, tribal governments have become more aggressive in policing the research done on their lands and have begun to develop their own or partner with other tribal research review boards. But the damage was done, because not only did this one study create havoc for Arizona, but it also had an impact on the way all tribes looked at research being conducted with their communities.

The failings here are numerous. Proper IRB protections were not followed and certainly tribal protections were not respected. Research is dependent upon an apprenticeship model whereby students learn by working with their senior research mentors; if the mentors do not follow proper procedure, the students will learn bad habits. Students and faculty alike should be aware of the rules regarding research on human participants. A truly informed consent means that the risks and benefits of the research are fully disclosed and that the participant understands the implications of participation. This is time-consuming and costly, but it is a requirement of the informed consent process. In this case, no students or investigators reported misconduct to the National Institutes of Health Office of Human Subjects Research.

On the surface, this project appeared to be a model community-based participatory research (CBPR) project. The community defined the problem of study, there were community partners, people were participating, and the tribal government was kept abreast of the study. Unfortunately, there was no transparency and all activities were not disclosed, even within the research team. This is a serious concern that some tribes have addressed by requiring that a member of the tribe be a key investigator on the studies.

## CONCLUSIONS

Each of these published case studies is evidence that programs fail despite good intentions. Lessons learned indicate that attention to political realities and the importance of communication is critical in a researcher-community relationship in order to avoid miscommunication or a breach of research ethics.

### Five Miles From Tomorrow

The story of suicide in Inuit territory (Shah 2000, Swenson 2001, AP 2001) is a lesson about the importance of respect. Shah could have demonstrated respect for the community by asking permission to print his story. Perhaps in so doing he would have received information that clarified his interpretation of the events. At the very least, he should have discussed the article with his supervising physician. *JAMA* could have done a better job of verifying the accuracy of the letter and could institute policies in the future that prevent such misinformation from being published. Finally, the institutions supervising Shah and Swenson could establish policies requiring medical students to take courses in bioethics and receive permission before writing about their experiences. Before they are allowed to disclose sensitive information about patients, supervisors should be sure that authors do not disclose any potential identifying information, including the name of the Native community, the family, and so forth. It is inappropriate to be a voice for a people who have not granted that privilege.

## Healthier Communities

The Healthier Communities (Wallerstein 1999) example illustrates that even an experienced community organizer and advocate for the principles of empowerment and community self-determination can make mistakes. Often the term CBPR is used to describe the project methodology, but the principles are not truly applied when implementing the research project. People of color frequently find themselves a token minority on an advisory board, and while a group may appear diverse, the minority participants hold no real power or decision-making responsibility. When working in Native communities, real involvement by the community requires more time and effort to build trust, an endeavor that may take years. Those in power—funders, researchers, and managers—need to evaluate their commitment to communities prior to initiating programs.

## Alaska Alcohol Project

Foulks reminds us that professional standards need to be established and negotiated with participants, sponsors, and third parties involved in projects. He reconfirms the need for full participation with the community and for paying particular attention to highly sensitive topics such as substance abuse and HIV/AIDS.

## Havasupai Versus Arizona Board of Regents

Finally, the Havasupai case is evidence of the need for transparency in partnerships, and the need for thoughtful and full disclosure of the consent process. It is a lesson that the values that Native communities hold dear are not necessarily the same as those of the research scientist; therefore, partnerships and transparency are critical to the success of the project.

## PARTING THOUGHTS

Native researchers are fully cognizant of the health disparities that exist in Native communities and are equally aware of the limited information available to help understand and address these disparities. Native researchers have sat in meetings in which scientists discussed the merits of research proposals, determining those that would be funded and those that would not, and have heard other scientists say that the Native population is too small for adequate statistical analysis to be meaningful. Native researchers are told that tribal sovereignty and demands for shared power make it too difficult to work with these communities. They also are told that the AIAN population constitute an insignificant portion of the population unworthy of federal funding despite the taxes that AIANs pay as individual citizens, tribal governments, and Native-owned businesses, and despite generations of historical government abuse and neglect. Comments such as these are inappropriate and limit equal access to health research, thereby limiting fair and equal treatment in health information, resources, or services that are derived from public research funding. Unfortunately, there are not enough NA health research scientists to cover the needs of NA communities. Well-trained and informed non-Native scientists should be part of the research program, and because race/ethnicity does not ensure that research will be conducted in a culturally competent manner, all researchers should be guided by the communities within which they wish to work.

Mistakes are often made by those with the best intentions. No one can foresee all the factors that may influence an outcome of an action. Native communities, after experiencing a history of unfulfilled promises, are often skeptical when approached by researchers. Open and frank discussions about the power that researchers possess or do not possess will improve relationships.

It is important for all investigators to draw upon the knowledge and experiences of tribal members and include them in a truly participatory fashion from the day a research idea is conceived to its ultimate evaluation and publication. The public health investigator should enter the community with an open heart and be prepared to be told that he or she does not belong or, if the particular culture so dictates, the community members may deliver their message of nonparticipation through passive resistance.

Researchers should not just take, but give back to the community. Resources should be shared, whether financial, technical, academic, or practical. And when researchers approach a community, they should plan to be there for the long haul. Relationship building takes a significant investment in time, energy, and other resources. Ultimately, a researcher should work with the community to find ways to translate his or her research findings into interventions and programs that make real changes to improve the well-being of Native peoples and their communities. "Good words" said Chief Joseph, Walla Band, Nez Perce, "do not last long unless they amount to something" (1879, p. 431).

## REFERENCES

Bommersbach J. 2008. Arizona's Broken Arrow: Did ASU Genetically Rape the Havasupai Tribe? *Phoenix Magazine*. November 2008:134–151.

Foulks EF. 1989. Misalliances in the Barrow alcohol study. *Am Indian Alsk Native Ment Health Res*. 2(3):7–17.

Joseph CY. 1879. An Indian's view of Indian affairs. *North Am Review*. 128(April):412–33.

Harmon A. 2010. Indian tribe wins fight to limit research of its DNA. *New York Times*. April 21, 2010:1–5. Available at: http://www.nytimes.com/2010/04/22/us/22dna.html/?th+&emc+th&pagewanted. Accessed April 21, 2010.

Shah S. 2000. A piece of my mind: five miles from tomorrow. *JAMA*. 284(15):1897–8.

Swenson MD. 2001. A story about suicide in the Arctic. *JAMA*. 286(8):919.

Tanner L. 2001. JAMA editors say they were duped. *Associated Press*. August 21, 2001.

Wallerstein N. 1999. Power between evaluator and community: research relationships within New Mexico's healthier communities. *Soc Sci Med*. 49(1):39–53.

# 10

# Developing Indigenous Research Policy: Some Key Considerations for Future Work

Doris M. Cook, PhD, MPH

## INTRODUCTION

Health status and the health disparities experienced by Indigenous people, including Canada's Indigenous population (Aboriginal peoples), are widely documented (Indian Health Service 2008, Reading and Nowgesic 2002, World Health Organization 2007). Addressing these disparities requires public health and clinical research initiatives that involve the active participation of Indigenous people (Chapter 3). Also supportive of the role of research in Indigenous health status is the Canadian Senate Standing Committee on Social Affairs, Science, and Technology. Volume six of its 2002 report states, "The Committee believes that research is perhaps the most important element that will help improve the health status of Aboriginal Canadians." Additionally, the World Health Organization asserts the importance of health information, including research. In order for health equity approaches to be successful, systematic health and demographic information on marginalized and disadvantaged groups, including Indigenous and tribal people, is needed (World Health Organization 2002). Concurrently, Indigenous and tribal people must be centrally involved in decisions affecting their health (United Nations 1994).

In addition to the recognition that interventions based on research results will ameliorate health disparities, there is a heightened awareness of the harmful and unethical research practices brought by researchers into Indigenous communities. The case of the Nuu-chah-nulth people from coastal British Columbia, Canada, whose blood was drawn for health research on arthritis and was used instead to establish ancestry, is an example of these practices (Wiwichar 2000). Similarly, the Havasupai people of Arizona report that unauthorized research was pursued using community member blood samples drawn for what they were told was research on diabetes but was then used to study schizophrenia, inbreeding, and population migration studies (Arizona Court of Appeals 2008). The result of breaches of research ethics such as this is intense suspicion of research and reluctance of Aboriginal people to participate in studies that may be beneficial to themselves and their communities (Arbour and Cook 2006). This issue is covered in much greater detail in Chapter 9.

This chapter presents the experience of the Canadian Institutes of Health Research (CIHR) in the development of research ethics policy for research involving Indigenous people, through examination of the history of the organization, extant research policy, and key considerations for the development of research policy. The intent is to provide practical guidance to those wishing to develop Indigenous policy by identifying process issues and factors that will facilitate policy development. This new approach to the policy development process, with its focus on stakeholder involvement, is equally relevant to the US Indigenous policy context. It provides an alternative implementation process for the 2000 US Presidential Executive Order 13175, which established a consultation policy that requires all federal agencies to establish regular and meaningful consultation and collaboration with Indian tribal officials in the development of federal policies that have tribal implications.

## CANADIAN INSTITUTES OF HEALTH RESEARCH AND RESEARCH PROTECTIONS

Since its creation in June 2000, CIHR has embraced an ambitious mission: to create and translate new knowledge to improve the health of Canadians, provide more effective health products and services, and strengthen Canada's healthcare system. As the premier funding agency for health research in Canada, CIHR provides stability and ensures an environment in which the research community can explore new scientific frontiers, nurture research talent of the highest caliber, foster partnerships and public engagement, generate exciting research breakthroughs, influence health policy and practice, commercialize new products and procedures, and improve health outcomes (Canadian Institutes of Health Research 2008).

As one of the 13 founding institutes of the CIHR, the Institute of Aboriginal People's Health (IAPH) is dedicated to leading an advanced research agenda in Aboriginal health. The five-year organizational plan and profile of the IAPH include support and promotion of health research that has a positive impact on the mental, physical, emotional, and spiritual health of Aboriginal people at all life stages (Institute of Aboriginal People's Health 2006). The IAPH is the only national Aboriginal or Indigenous health institute in the world, devoted to the advancement of holistic and multidisciplinary health research for Indigenous people.

In 1998, the *Tri-Council Policy Statement: Ethical Conduct for Research Involving Humans* (TCPS) was formally adopted by Canada's three federal research granting agencies: (1) the Medical Research Council (now CIHR), (2) the Natural Sciences and Engineering Research Council, and (3) the Social Sciences and Humanities Research Council. The new policy was intended to express "the continuing commitment by the three Councils to the people of Canada, to promote the ethical conduct of research involving human subjects" (Canadian Institutes of Health Research, Natural Sciences and Engineering Research Council, Social Sciences and Humanities Research Council 1998). The policy, expressed in the form of guidelines for researchers, is intended to protect the health, safety, and human rights of individual research participants. While adherence to the guidelines is not a regulatory requirement and compliance is voluntary, the funding councils only consider funding for researchers and institutions that certify compliance with the policy.

Section six of the TCPS was intended to focus on research involving Aboriginal peoples. Since the adoption of the policy, there has been a general acknowledgment that section six required further development. In fact, a statement indicating that insufficient consultation had taken place during the development of the policy was included in a preamble to section six (Canadian Institutes of Health Research, Natural Sciences and Engineering Research

Council, Social Sciences and Humanities Research Council 1998). As a result, section six is considered to be a set of best practices and is inconsistent with the more directive tone of the remainder of the policy.

Since 1998, the research guidelines have been implemented within the wider research community; however, Aboriginal participants and their respective communities lacked adequate protections. Communities could be placed at risk when members participated in research designed to produce information about the community. The autonomy and collective decision-making of Aboriginal communities were not addressed in the research guidelines, which left communities feeling vulnerable. Other countries with significant Indigenous populations such as Australia and New Zealand have successfully developed Indigenous-specific research guidelines (Australian Institute of Aboriginal and Torres Strait Islander Studies 2000, Health Research Council of New Zealand 2008). Previous Canadian attempts to develop Aboriginal research guidelines were not successful and did not have either the involvement of Aboriginal people in the process to ensure policy relevance and appropriateness or a sufficient understanding of Aboriginal culture and values surrounding research. The absence of a systematic approach involving Aboriginal peoples both in the consultations and management of the policy development has been one of the main reasons for unsuccessful policy development. Additionally, the lack of attention to the dynamics involved in management of the policy development process may have adversely affected the successful development and implementation of Indigenous policy initiatives.

Canada's decision in 2000 to establish an institute (IAPH) devoted to the advancement of Indigenous health research, as a part of CIHR, responded not only to its own domestic health disparities but also to the United Nations position on the need for continued improvements in the health of Indigenous peoples (United Nations High Commissioner for Human Rights Commission 1994). The expected long-term outcome of CIHR-funded health research is to improve the health of Aboriginal people. The CIHR considers the active participation of Aboriginal communities integral to the research process (Institute of Aboriginal People's Health 2006). To respond to this new opportunity for involvement in decision-making and setting the Aboriginal research agenda, stakeholders would have to be involved in the development of research guidelines that would ensure culturally competent research that is protective of the health, safety, and human rights of Aboriginal people, while at the same time promoting research. There is a limited body of North American literature on Indigenous policy development and the need for Indigenous participation, such as Cobin and Hsu (1998) and Cornell (2004), and therefore, practical guidance on the approach or management of Indigenous policy development initiatives remains underdeveloped.

In the context of managing an advisory body to provide advice and steering for the development of policy, team building is thought to be essential. Team building is a method designed to help teams operate more effectively by improving internal communication and problem-solving skills. Understanding the dynamics of team work and those factors that facilitate or impede its functioning is essential to better understanding of project management in the Indigenous policy development context. The work of Cobin and Hsu (1998) focuses on the driving and restraining forces that bear on the establishment and maintenance of partnerships involving traditional medicine. Expanding the application of those forces and team building to the management and policy development arena facilitates the development of a framework that could be useful in the management of Indigenous projects. This Aboriginal research policy development initiative can provide practical guidance to organizations wishing to develop Indigenous policy in a collaborative and inclusive fashion by identifying factors that will facilitate or impede policy development in the Indigenous context.

## KEY CONSIDERATIONS FOR POLICY DEVELOPMENT

Public consultations during the development of public policy have become de rigueur for governmental agencies. The public has expectations to be consulted as a part of ongoing stakeholder engagement as policy is being discussed and developed; consultations also serve as a method of accountability for publicly funded services (Gregory 2003). Stakeholder consultation should be seen not only as a requirement but also as insurance that public policy reflects the needs of stakeholders. Two of the greatest challenges to the development of Indigenous policy are (1) to ensure that the policy meets the needs of the Indigenous population and is culturally appropriate and (2) that the policy development process engages stakeholders to ensure its ongoing relevancy.

Over the long term, successful organization performance requires the establishment of a mutually satisfactory relationship with a broad range of stakeholders. The establishment of a trust relationship with stakeholders is an essential antecedent to collaborative planning (Petersen et al. 2005). Similarly, Ryan and Buchholtz (2001) explored a trust/risk decision-making model in the context of shareholder investment decisions, concluding that trust is an antecedent to risk evaluation in shareholder decision-making. The Indigenous community has long considered trust as an essential element of relationships with bodies external to the community. Supporting this premise is a limited body of evidence in Indigenous and international literature emphasizing the importance of stakeholder trust and involvement in health policy development (World Health Organization 2002, Cobin and Hsu 1998, Cornell 2004). Thus, the management of stakeholder relations is a critical factor for successful development of Indigenous policy.

Throughout the course of creating a committee to provide advice and project steering, management is a key consideration. Delta (2006) defines management as the process of setting and achieving the goals of the organization: planning, organizing, directing (or leading), and controlling. These managerial functions are generally carried out in the context of supervising employees or teams empowered to establish their objectives, make decisions about how to achieve those objectives, undertake the tasks required to meet them, and be accountable for their results. Empowerment is the delegation of authority to an individual or team and includes autonomy, trust, and encouragement to make the decisions necessary to accomplish the job. The efficacy of team decision-making outcomes is a critical measure of management performance (Wagner and Hollenbeck 1998).

The issues of stakeholder consultations, trust relationships with stakeholders, and project management including group dynamics are concerned with the impact of certain factors such as communications, resources, cultural competency, sensitivity, and diversity of beliefs on the management process. It is important to consider how individual characteristics including cultural factors affect selection of members of the project advisory committee as well as how these factors may facilitate or hinder group processes. Based on the previous discussion, broad-based stakeholder support and engagement and active involvement are thought to be central factors of successful Indigenous policy development.

## THE POLICY DEVELOPMENT PROCESS

Prior to initiating the guidelines development project, the Aboriginal community voiced a number of concerns with research that had been previously conducted within their communities. Communities saw research being done for reasons that benefited researchers such as career advancement, advanced degrees, and publications rather than research that might be of community benefit. In addition, communities were concerned with the secondary use of data and samples, such as in the Nuu-chah-nulth case, and wanted a greater degree of control and involvement with research conducted in their communities.

In 2004, CIHR initiated a project to develop Aboriginal-specific health research guidelines. The project was designed to set ground rules that would promote mutually beneficial research that respected Aboriginal culture and values and addressed the needs of researchers for clear guidance when undertaking research involving Aboriginal peoples. The project also sought to promote respectful partnerships between researchers and communities in health research and ethics review. Developing culturally appropriate guidelines that promote good research is what the agency needs for accountability and credibility; ongoing engagement as partners and participation in the review process helps ensures respect for self-determination, community processes and priorities, and community requests for involvement.

An advisory committee, the Aboriginal Ethics Working Group (AEWG), was established in March 2004 to provide technical and scientific advice and support for the development of ethics guidelines for health research. The composition of the AEWG ensured diverse citizen engagement in this issue and reflected a broad range of relevant disciplines and interests, such as the Aboriginal community, Indigenous studies, anthropology, ethics, law, medicine, public health, and the natural and social sciences. The majority of the members of the AEWG are Aboriginal peoples (Indians, Inuit, and Métis) from First Nations, Northern, rural, and urban communities.

The AEWG met to deliberate, discuss, and draft the guidelines over the course of two years. A series of commissioned background papers informed the deliberations of the AEWG. The background papers explored issues that have been causing difficulty for researchers and communities alike, such as community or group consent and how to conduct ethical research in urban Aboriginal environments. The group adopted a hands-on approach to guideline development and adopted ethical principles to guide its own work. The first principles adopted by the group included respect for Aboriginal values, knowledge, methodologies, and decision-making processes as well as a commitment to an inclusive, participatory process that engages Aboriginal and research communities. There was an early recognition that the knowledge, expertise, and resources of the community are often key to successful research and that research partnerships based on mutual trust and respect lead to better research and a more positive relationship with communities and individuals that are affected by the research.

A comprehensive nation-wide strategy for consultation with Aboriginal communities, researchers and institutions was built on the Aboriginal Capacity and Development Research Environment (ACADRE) network, an initiative of the CIHR-Institute for Aboriginal People's Health. The ACADRE network was a unique academically based resource with links to academic research communities and partnerships with regional First Nations, Inuit, and Métis communities. Proposals for research ethics collaboration were accepted from the ACADRE centres; each proposal was unique to the center. Early ACADRE work focused on work with communities to translate traditional values and

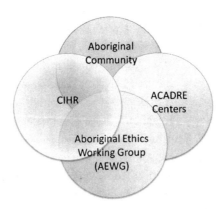

Figure 10.1. Pictorial representation of the partnership between the Aboriginal community, academic research community, project advisory committee, and Canadian Institutes of Health Research (CIHR) for the guidelines development project.

ethics into guidance for health researchers, which formed the foundation for the guidelines (Figure 10.1). The first draft of research guidelines was completed in May 2005.

Initial vetting of the draft guidelines took place through the ACADRE network and their community partners to determine cultural appropriateness and acceptability. The wider academic community was then invited to provide commentary and feedback. Consultations and vetting throughout Aboriginal and research communities began in fall 2005 and continued through March 2006; the ACADRE network conducted these sessions as a part of their proposals for collaboration. Additionally, the CIHR Ethics Office along with the National Council on Ethics in Human Research conducted workshops and consultations with Aboriginal communities, researchers, and institutional research ethics board members to obtain feedback on the draft guidelines. The high level of interest by the Aboriginal and research communities, and request for additional workshops and consultations, resulted in two timeline extensions for feedback. The guidelines were electronically posted by CIHR and its partners to ensure awareness of the guidelines and solicit commentary prior to its final revision. This approach contributed to achieving a workable balance for the multiple, diverse perspectives expressed on issues such as community authority and jurisdiction, and is seen as a positive, productive indicator and educative contribution to research ethics.

## THE GUIDELINES: OPERATIONALIZING RESPECT FOR COMMUNITIES

The Guidelines for Health Research Involving Aboriginal People were formally adopted by the CIHR Governing Council in March 2007 and serve as a model for both the protection of the health, safety, and human rights of Indigenous research participants and the development of Indigenous policy initiatives (Canadian Institutes of Health Research 2008). The guidelines are designed to facilitate the ethical conduct of research involving Aboriginal peoples, and the intent is to promote health through research in keeping with Indigenous values and traditions. Table 10.1 provides a list of the substantive principles that are embodied within the guidelines.

**Table 10.1. Substantive Principles for Ethically Sound Health Research**

- Cultural responsibilities, traditional knowledge, and community protocols
- Community jurisdiction and approval
- Research partnership methodology
- Community and individual consent
- Confidentiality and privacy
- Inclusion of Indigenous knowledge in research
- Protection of Indigenous knowledge and culture
- Benefit sharing and capacity development
- Cultural protocol, language, and communication
- Data collection, storage, management, secondary use, and data transfer to third parties
- Collection, storage, and management of biological samples
- Interpretation of results and due credit
- Memorandum of understanding and research agreements, including a best practices model research agreement
- Protocol procedures in schematic flow chart form (a step-by-step process for establishing research partnerships and obtaining ethics approval)

Section 1.2 includes the following passage, which underlies the rationale for the guidelines:

Some Aboriginal communities manage and control matters dealing with health. As part of this control, the community may choose to be a full participant in any

- Research conducted within or about it;
- Community consent process.

Consequently, researchers will need to meet those communities' standards and recognize their authority over such research.

Research agreements should be negotiated and formalized with the appropriate community authority before research is commenced. Aboriginal communities may have their own research ethics guidelines and processes, including research ethics boards.

Although individual consent is essential, Aboriginal social norms and values tend to be organized around an operative principle of collective Aboriginal knowledge, ownership and decision-making. This is one of the reasons why the notion of community consent is so important in research involving Aboriginal people. Thus, an Aboriginal community is entitled to decide whether a research project is in the best interest of the community (community consent) as a precondition to the researcher seeking individual consent from community members (Canadian Institutes of Health Research 2008).

Thus, the basis for respectful engagement of communities was established. The negotiation of a research agreement prior to the initiation of a research initiative is a central tenet of the guidelines. The guidelines provide the following discussion on the research agreement:

> The agreement should detail issues of data ownership, use and interpretation/analysis, rights to intellectual property (if appropriate), and expectations regarding process, content and authorship of publications, with identified mechanisms for dealing with conflicting interpretations or inappropriate use of the data. There should be prior agreement on the respective roles of the parties, desired outcomes, measures of validity, control over the use of data, funding and the dissemination of research findings (Canadian Institutes of Health Research 2008).

## CONCLUSIONS

Aboriginal stakeholder involvement in policy development through representation on the project advisory committee and through public consultations was found to be critical to early success and progress on the CIHR initiative to develop sound Aboriginal research policy. Aboriginal involvement was essential to understand the cultural dynamics and problems experienced by communities involved in research. Ongoing consultations reaffirmed the appropriateness of the overall strategy and ensured that an acceptable and workable policy was developed. Respectful engagement of the Aboriginal community and the development of partnerships in policy development helped to build trust among partners and currently are facilitating the dismantling of barriers to community participation in beneficial research. Finally, attention to management of the policy development process including planning, organizing, and leading the project was important to successful policy development.

With the adoption of the guidelines, institutional and researcher compliance with the new guidelines is a requirement for receipt of CIHR grants and awards. In December 2010, a revised TCPS that includes a chapter for research involving Aboriginal peoples was adopted by Canada's three research funding agencies. The CIHR Web site includes the following statement:

> The inclusion of Chapter 9 in the revised TCPS would not have been possible without previous work undertaken by CIHR and its Aboriginal partners to create the former CIHR policy: Guidelines for Health Research Involving Aboriginal People. These Guidelines, on which the new chapter of TCPS is based, have been rightfully acknowledged both nationally and internationally, not only for the rigor of their content, but also for the collaborative approach by which they were developed (Canadian Institutes of Health Research 2010, Canadian Institutes of Health Research 2011, Cook 2007).

## ACKNOWLEDGMENTS

This chapter is an expansion of a paper prepared and presented at the Global Forum on Health Research's Forum 10, Cairo, Egypt, October 29-November 2, 2006, entitled, "The Importance of Ethically Sound Health Research to Improvements in Aboriginal Health."

## REFERENCES

Arbour L, Cook D. 2006. DNA on loan: issues to consider when carrying out genetic research with Aboriginal families and communities. *Community Genet.* 9:153–160.

Arizona Court of Appeals. 2008. *Opinion Havasupai Tribe V. Arizona Board of Regents and Therese Ann Markow.* Available at: http://www.azcourts.gov/Portals/0/OpinionFiles/Div1/2008/1%20CA-CV%2007-0454.PDF. Accessed July 26, 2013.

Australian Institute of Aboriginal and Torres Strait Islander Studies. 2000. *Guidelines for Ethical Research in Indigenous Studies.* Available at: http://www.aiatsis.gov.au/research/docs/ethics.pdf. Accessed July 20, 2013.

Canadian Institutes of Health Research. 2008. *Annual Report 2007–2008*. Ottawa, ON: Canadian Institutes of Health Research.

Canadian Institutes of Health Research. 2011. Ethics of Health Research Involving First Nations, Inuit and Metis People. Available at: http://www.cihr.ca/e/29339.html. Accessed July 20, 2013.

Canadian Institutes of Health Research, Natural Sciences and Engineering Research Council, & Social Sciences and Humanities Research Council. 1998. Tri Council Policy Statement: Ethical Conduct for Research Involving Humans. Available at: http://www. pre.ethics.gc.ca/eng/archives/tcps-eptc/Default. Accessed September 30, 2013.

Canadian Institutes of Health Research, Natural Sciences and Engineering Research Council of Canada, and Social Sciences and Humanities Research Council of Canada. 2010. *Tri-Council Policy Statement: Ethical Conduct for Research Involving Humans, December 2010*. Available at: http://www.pre.ethics.gc.ca/pdf/eng/tcps2/ TCPS_2_FINAL_Web.pdf. Accessed July 20, 2013.

Canadian Senate Standing Committee on Social Affairs. 2002. Science and Technology Report. Vol. 6. Available at: http://www.parl.gc.ca/content/sen/committee/371/soci/rep/ repjan01vol2-e.pdf. Accessed July 20, 2013.

Cobin G, Hsu L. 1998. *The Partnership of Traditional Navajo Medicine and Biomedical Health Care Practices at the Chinle Comprehensive Care Facility*. Cambridge, MA: Harvard University, JFK School of Government. Available at: http://hpaied.org/images/ resources/publibrary/PRS98-24.pdf. Accessed September 30, 2013.

Cook D. 2007. CIHR's new guidelines for Aboriginal health research: setting the ground rules. *Canadian J Diabetes*. 31:198–199.

Cornell S. 2004. *Power to the People: The North American Experience of Empowering Indigenous Communities* [Opinion]. Available at: http://www.onlineopinion.com.au/ view.asp?article=2605. Accessed July 20, 2013.

Delta Publishing. 2006. *Understanding and Managing Organizational Behavior*. Available at: http://www.apexcpe.com/Publications/471001.pdf. Accessed July 26, 2013.

Gregory A. 2003. The ethics of engagement in the UK public sector: A case in point. *J Commun Mgmt*. 8(1):83–94.

Health Research Council of New Zealand. 2008. *Guidelines for Researchers on Health Research Involving Māori*. Available at: http://www.hrc.govt.nz/sites/default/files/

Guidelines%20for%20HR%20on%20Maori-%20Jul10%20revised%20for%20Te%20Ara
%20Tika%20v2%20FINAL%5B1%5D.pdf Accessed July 26, 2013.

Indian Health Service. 2008. *IHS Fact Sheet: Year 2008 Profile*. Available at: http://www.ihs.gov/PublicAffairs/IHSBrochure/Profile08.asp. Accessed March 20, 2012.

Institute of Aboriginal People's Health. 2006. *Five-Year Strategic Plan: 2006 to 2011*. Available at: http://www.cihr-irsc.gc.ca/e/9188.html. Accessed July 20, 2013.

Petersen KJ, Ragatz GL, Monczka RM. 2005. An examination of collaborative planning effectiveness and supply chain performance. *J Supply Chain Mgmt*. 41(2):14–25.

Reading J, Nowgesic E. 2002. Improving the health of future generations: the Canadian Institutes of Health Research Institute of Aboriginal Peoples' Health. *Am J Public Health*. 92(9):1396–1400.

Ryan LV, Buchholtz AK. 2001. Trust, risk and shareholder decision making: an investor perspective on corporate governance. *Business Ethics Quarterly*. 11(1):177–193.

United Nations High Commissioner for Human Rights Commission. 1994. *Draft United Nations Declaration on the rights of Indigenous peoples, United Nations*. Available at: http://www.ohchr.org/EN/Issues/IPeoples/Pages/WGDraftDeclaration.aspx. Accessed March 20, 2012.

Wagner J, Hollenbeck J. 1998. *Organizational Behavior: Securing Competitive Advantage*. Upper Saddle River, New Jersey: Prentice Hall.

Wiwichar D. September 2000. Bad blood. *Ha-Shilth-Sa*. p. 21.

World Health Organization. 2002. *International Decade of the World's Indigenous People: Report by the Secretariat, World Health Organization*. Available at: http://www.who.int/hhr/activities/indigenous_peoples/International_decade_indigenous_peopleWHA55_35.pdf. Accessed September 30, 2013.

World Health Organization. 2007. *The Health of Indigenous Peoples: Fact Sheet*. Available at: http://www.who.int/hhr/Fact%20Sheet%20Indigenous%20Health%20Nov%202007%20Final%20ENG.pdf. Accessed July 20, 2013.

# 11

# Ethics of Biospecimen Research

Francine C. Gachupin, PhD, MPH, CIP, and William L. Freeman, MD, MPH, CIP

## INTRODUCTION

> The take-home message is that we must do 'culturally competent' research, research that respects the Indigenous community's beliefs, their desire for self-determination, their desire to benefit from the research, and their wish to retain intellectual property rights and ownership of samples of DNA, issues and body fluids (McInnes 2011, p. 255).

The protection of human participants in research within the United States is guided by federal regulations (US Department of Health and Human Services [DHHS] 2011, 2012), with several limitations that have significant implications for tribal peoples. First, the federal regulations focus on protection of individuals participating in research and do not extend protections to families or to communities. This is important because according to the 2010 US Census, approximately 33% of American Indian and Alaska Native (AIAN) respondents (those who marked their race as American Indian and Alaska Native alone) reported their residence within American Indian areas or Alaska Native village statistical areas (Norris et al. 2012). For researchers working with these Native peoples, approval for projects also requires tribal review and approval. Second, although research involving biological specimens (such as genetics) has made unprecedented advances both as a tool and a science in medical and scientific applications, federal regulations lag behind. At present, no comprehensive law protects genetic privacy and there exists no overarching federal or industry guidelines for commercial genetic testing (Spector-Bagdady 2013).

Federal regulations that currently exist to protect individuals involved in research do not extend to protection of their culture, tradition, or religion. In this chapter we underscore the need to consider Native holistic world views, established disease or illness explanations, and the continuum from present life to the afterlife when engaging Native people in research (Freeman and Gachupin, unpublished manuscript, 2013). Many people believe that researchers retain ethical obligations to participants beyond the time the participants donate their biospecimens.

This chapter presents an overview of regulations specific to the use of biospecimens in research and outlines the ethical obligations of the researcher given that protections are limited. An overview of topics to consider when engaging tribal entities in research with biospecimens is presented to provide understanding and guidance to those wishing to facilitate or develop Indigenous policy by identifying risks, potential harm, and responsibilities.

## BIOSPECIMEN RESEARCH IN INDIAN COUNTRY: AN EXAMPLE

Within Indian country there is great concern about genetic research because some researchers have used specimens for use not authorized by tribes and others have shared samples with colleagues and students without explicit approval from tribes (Harmon 2010a, Harmon 2010b, Wiwchar 2004, Wiwchar nd; Romero et al., personal communication, 2000). Even with these very real concerns, several tribes have approved genetic studies focused on heart disease, an important area of research since cardiovascular disease is the leading cause of death among AIAN persons (Barnes et al. 2010, Schiller et al. 2012, Kochanek et al. 2011, DHHS 2008). One study, the Strong Heart Study (SHS), has been funded by the National Heart, Lung, and Blood Institute (NHLBI) since October 1, 1988. The SHS, the largest epidemiologic study of American Indians ever undertaken, is designed to estimate cardiovascular disease mortality and morbidity and the prevalence of known and suspected cardiovascular disease risk factors (Ali et al. 2001). The SHS includes 13 American Indian tribes and communities in four states: seven tribes from southwestern Oklahoma (Apache, Caddo, Comanche, Delaware, Fort Sill Apache, Kiowa, and Wichita), three tribes from Arizona (Gila River and Salt

River Pima/Maricopa, and Akchin Pima/Papago), and three Sioux Tribes from South/North Dakota (Oglala Sioux, Cheyenne River Sioux, and Spirit Lake Communities).

The SHS was completed in phases and in 1996, Phases III, IV, and V expanded to investigate the heritability of cardiovascular disease and its risk factors (including diabetes and obesity) and to localize genes that contribute to cardiovascular disease risk (NHLBI 2006). The component of the SHS dedicated to assessing the genetic contributions to cardiovascular disease became known as the Strong Heart Family Study (SHFS), and is the only one of its kind. The SHFS enrolled 3,800 family members across the different sites. Investigators found evidence for a gene influencing weight and body mass index, a gene influencing insulin and lean body mass, and a region influencing blood pressure differently between men and women (Franceschini et al. 2008, Almasy et al. 2007, Diego et al. 2006, North et al. 2005).

As would be expected for a multicenter national study, the coordination of the SHS was no small feat. The SHS Web site has links to invaluable information and includes: a coronary heart disease risk calculator, diabetes risk calculator, community education brochures, newsletters, operations manual, forms, data request policy, publications list, descriptions of the respective phases, and announcements (NHLBI 2006). The SHS experience provides unparalleled amounts of data to tribes and investigators alike on cardiovascular disease morbidity and mortality specific to select American Indian tribes, a large-scale epidemiologic study in Indian country, and genetics research among many American Indian tribes.

One has to wonder what the fate of the SHS would have been if the research began a decade later. It is fortunate that such important study predated several national and international activities that caused concern among many Indigenous populations from around the world regarding genetic research, including the Human Genome Diversity Project (Cavalli-Sforza 2005), the Kennewick Man (Burke Museum of Natural History and Culture 2013), and the Yanomami of the Amazon (Tierney 2002).

## CURRENT REGULATIONS FOR BIOSPECIMEN USE RESEARCH

By regulations, all human participant research conducted in facilities or with staff or resources funded through federal sources must be approved by an institutional review board (IRB; DHHS 2011, 2012). It is the responsibility of each investigator to abide by institutional requirements and to plan research well in advance to fulfill other requirements such as tribal review and approval and approval by an Indian Health Service or tribal IRB (DHHS 2013, Gachupin 2012). For research involving biological specimens, IRB oversight may not apply if samples are de-identified or are from decedents. IRB regulations apply only to research involving living human participants.

Biological samples do originate from individuals and it is the investigator's responsibility to ensure that consent is truly informed; that is, that individuals understand the extent of the use of their biological specimens, whether the samples are identifiable, whether they can be accessed at a later time for removal or destruction, who has access to the samples, and whether the samples can and will be used for future research or by other researchers.

The current federal regulations include guidance from the Office for Human Research Protections (OHRP) for 45 Code of Federal Regulations (CFR) 46; the US Food and Drug Administration (FDA) for 21 CFR parts 812, 50, 56; and the Health Insurance Portability and Accountability Act (HIPAA). OHRP's 45 CFR 46, subpart A, does permit consent of participants to future unspecified research (DHHS 2009). FDA's 21 CFR part 812 outlines responsibilities when human specimens are used for in vitro diagnostic device studies that utilize "leftover" biospecimens (DHHS 2006, 2012). HIPAA requires that each authorization by the patient for release of protected health information include a specific research purpose (DHHS 2003). HIPAA was very recently modified under the Health Information Technology for Economic and Clinical Health Act (HITECH) and the Genetic Information Nondiscrimination Act (GINA) to strengthen the privacy and security protection for individuals' health information (HITECH) and privacy protections for genetic information (GINA; DHHS 2013). The HITECH Act, enacted as part of the American Recovery and Reinvestment Act of 2009, was signed into law on February 17, 2009, to promote the adoption and meaningful use of health information technology. Subtitle D of the HITECH Act addresses the privacy and security concerns associated with the electronic transmission of health information, in part, through several provisions that strengthen the civil and criminal enforcement of HIPAA (DHHS 2009). Title II of GINA prohibits discrimination against employees or applicants because of genetic information. The Departments of Labor, Health and Human Services, and Treasury have responsibility for issuing regulations for Title I of GINA, which addresses the use of genetic information in health insurance (US Equal Opportunity and Employment Commission 2009).

In addition to federal regulations, it is important to ensure compliance with state-specific genetic privacy statutes (National Congress of State Legislatures 2009). For example, in Alaska genetic information is explicitly defined as personal property, which in turn extends personal property rights to DNA samples. In New Mexico, personal access to genetic information is required. Both Alaska and New Mexico require consent to perform or require genetic tests, obtain or access genetic information, retain genetic information, and disclose genetic information (National Congress of State Legislatures 2009).

Because the regulations can be quite daunting and confusing, IRB or agency staff members should be sought during the research development phase to answer questions and provide additional guidance. Other resources are available to researchers—for example, the National Cancer Institute (NCI) has produced a very helpful guide entitled "NCI Best Practices for Biospecimen Resources" (DHHS 2007).

Within an academic university setting, in addition to the IRB there may be several other required levels of clearance and approval. For example, a project with biospecimens may require biosafety and biosecurity committee review; tissue repository committee clearance; radiation, chemical, and biological safety committee clearance; export control review; conflict of interest clearance; and scientific advisory committee review and approval. Furthermore, the sequence in receiving clearance and approval is important to follow. At the University of New Mexico, for example, the Institutional Biosafety Committee's approval is required prior to the IRB's review for research involving select hazardous agents such as rDNA (University of New Mexico 2013).

The above guidance forms the basis of the "right way" to do research involving biological specimens. The remaining sections of this chapter will focus on forming the basis of conducting ethical research with Indigenous populations. Ethics is defined as "dealing with what is good and bad and with moral duty and obligation" (Encyclopaedia Britannica Company 2013).

## CONSIDERATIONS WHEN ENGAGING TRIBES IN RESEARCH INVOLVING BIOSPECIMENS

Most American Indians and Alaska Natives have an established relationship with their physical environment and either a written or oral understanding of their origin as a people. There are established intra- and inter-tribal relationships and understandings of familial relationships that may or may not be related to heredity. For many Native people, there are established explanations for disease and illness and the belief that the soul of a person transcends from the physical body to the spiritual realm upon death. The worldview of many Native peoples does not separate the physical from the spiritual—all of these are important to consider when addressing custodianship and ownership issues of biological specimens.

Native peoples become extremely concerned when their established relationship with the physical environment or their understandings of their origin as a people is threatened. Potential harms at the community level include biologic determinism in and by public policy—for example, determining group membership by whether or not individuals possess "Indian markers." Other potential harms include decreased political or social status in society and having research results challenge a community's understanding of who they are and where they came from (Freeman and Gachupin, unpublished manuscript, 2013).

Concerns abound when there are challenges to an individual or group's understanding of family dynamics (Freeman and Gachupin, unpublished manuscript, 2013). Potential harms include misattributed paternity and misattributed non-relationship—for example, an adoption with later marriage of individuals who turn out to be close relatives. In family studies it is also important to anticipate altered feelings of self—for example, survivor guilt if the test is negative and fear of the future if the test is positive. Additionally, recruitment into a family study can create intra-family coercion and discord. As with all clinical trials, it is imperative to ensure understanding of study objectives and not to raise expectations about receiving more benefit from the research than the research and researcher can give (i.e., therapeutic misconception).

As mentioned previously, the worldview of many Native peoples does not separate the physical from the spiritual; as such, it causes great dignitary harm to communities and individuals when biological specimens are placed in a repository. This becomes even more harmful when the specimens are placed in repositories without explicit knowledge and approval. It is equally important to respect the requests of tribes in reference to establishment of immortal cell lines, maintaining systems to identify samples if withdrawal or destruction is expected, and contacting of individuals or communities if reconsenting for use of samples for subsequent use is required or requested.

In order to respectfully work with AIAN persons, it is important to recognize and work within boundaries of individual and community worldviews. It is also imperative to recognize that in some tribal communities it is a cultural norm to have the community or family make decisions for individuals and that these decisions trump individual autonomy. As researchers work in tribal communities, it is important to be aware of competing interests and understand the disease challenges faced by AIAN persons. A particular research focus or question of interest may not be shared by tribes; to ensure the highest level of participation by Native communities, it is recommended to conduct research on topics of priority to tribes and to involve them from the onset of project design and development.

Science is a powerful tool for progress against disease; both individuals and communities can promote good science to improve health and well-being. A responsible investigator working with AIAN persons should adhere to the following basic tenets: respect for tribal culture and traditions; respect for tribal sovereignty and self-determination; respect for concerns and opinions of community; respect for local research priorities and needs; respect for individuals, families, and communities; respect for human participants' rights and dignity; respect for a tribe's right to decline participation; respect for the autonomy and decisions of the tribe; taking time to demystify research; taking time to be accessible; and providing feedback and findings in a timely manner (Romero and Kanade 2000).

## RESOURCES FOR ADDITIONAL GUIDANCE ON BIOSPECIMEN USE RESEARCH

In November 2009, President Obama established the Presidential Commission for the Study of Bioethical Issues (2013). The commission is tasked to advise the president on ethical issues arising from advances in biomedicine and related areas of science and technology. In the relatively short existence of the commission, four reports have already been released to provide recommenda-tions: (1) *New Directions, The Ethics of Synthetic Biology and Emerging Technologies*, released on December 16, 2010; (2) *"Ethically Impossible" STD Research in Guatemala from 1946 to 1948*, released on September 13, 2011; (3) *Moral Science: Protecting Participants in Human Subjects Research*, released on December 15, 2011; and (4) *Privacy and Progress in Whole Genome Sequencing*, released on October 2, 2012 (DHHS 2013). The reports exemplify policies and practices that are being put forward to ensure that scientific research, healthcare delivery, and technological innovation are conducted in a socially and ethically responsible manner.

In 2012, the National Congress of American Indians (NCAI) created an American Indian & Alaska Native Genetics Resource Center to provide tools and information to tribes to make informed decisions about genetic research (NCAI 2009). In the previous chapter, Dr. Cook provided background on the 2007 *CIHR Guidelines for Health Research Involving Aboriginal People*, the current tri-council policy on ethical conduct for research involving humans (Government of Canada 1998, 2007), and other Indigenous policies at the international level (United Nations 2007, Australian Institute of Aboriginal and Torres Strait Islander Studies 2011, Health Research Council of New Zealand 2010).

## LIMITATIONS IN BIOSPECIMEN RESEARCH GUIDANCE AND REGULATIONS

There are limitations in AIAN and Indigenous biospecimen research guidance and regulations that need to be recognized and hopefully, remedied, so that policies and protections will be provided at the highest levels for Indigenous peoples. In the United States we do not have research guidelines and a code of ethics specific to AIAN individuals and communities at the federal agency (e.g., the Secretary's Advisory Committee on Human Research Protections, which makes recommendations to the Office for Human Research Protections), national association, or the peer-reviewed journal level (to ensure that published articles are in compliance with tribal review, clearance, and approval for publication). Even within existing regulations, protections for AIAN persons are deficient. For example, 45 CFR 46 does not include any requirements for tribal approval for studies occurring on reservations. Some progress is being made, however; in July 2011, the US Department of Health and Human Services made available to the public an opportunity to comment on various ways to enhance regulations overseeing research on human participants, an opportune time to influence policy change (2011).

Other limitations in biospecimen research guidance and regulation include insufficient detail and overview of policies and regulations regarding incidental findings, data use agreements, materials use agreements, or intellectual property—all important subjects in their own rights. Researchers are encouraged to explore these additional topics.

## SUMMARY

This chapter offers an overview of an existing genetic study with Native people, provides background on existing regulations and guidance, outlines tribe-specific considerations for researchers when engaging Native American communities and tribal nations in biospecimen research, and supplies resources throughout for reference and background. Finally, we propose a foundation on which to build biospecimen research in a respectful manner toward Native peoples.

## REFERENCES

Ali T, Jarvis B, O'Leary M. 2001. *M. Strong Heart Study Data Book, A Report to American Indian Communities*. Rockville, MD: National Institute of Health, National Heart, Lung and Blood Institute, Division of Epidemiology and Clinical Applications. NIH Publication No. 01-3285.

Almasy L, Goring HH, Diego V, et al. 2007. A novel obesity locus on chromosome 4q: the Strong Heart Family Study. *Obesity*. 15(7):1741-8.

Australian Institute of Aboriginal and Torres Strait Islander Studies. 2011. *Guidelines for Ethical Research in Australian Indigenous Studies*. Available at: http://www.aiatsis. gov.au/research/docs/ethics.pdf. Accessed March 7, 2013.

Barnes PM, Adams PF, Powell-Griner E. 2010. *Health Characteristics of the American Indian or Alaska Native Adult Population: United States, 2004–2008*. Available at: http://www.cdc.gov/nchs/data/nhsr/nhsr020.pdf. Accessed March 3, 2013.

Burke Museum of Natural History and Culture, University of Washington, Seattle. 2013. *Kennewick Man.* Available at: http://www.burkemuseum.org/kman. Accessed March 5, 2013.

Canadian Institutes of Health Research. 2007. *CIHR Guidelines for Health Research Involving Aboriginal People.* Available at: http://www.cihr-irsc.gc.ca/e/29134.html. Accessed March 7, 2013.

Canadian Government, Canadian Institutes of Health Research, Natural Sciences and Engineering Research Council, and Social Sciences and Humanities Research Council. 2010. *Tri-Council Policy Statement: Ethical Conduct for Research Involving Humans.* Available at: http://www.pre.ethics.gc.ca/eng/policy-politique/initiatives/tcps2-eptc2/ Default. Accessed March 7, 2013.

Cavalli-Sforza LL. 2005. The Human Genome Diversity Project: past, present and future. *Nature Reviews Genetics.* 6:333–340.

Diego VP, Goring HH, Cole SA, et al. 2006. Fasting insulin and obesity-related phenotypes are linked to chromosome 2p: the Strong Heart Family Study. *Diabetes.* 55(6):1874–8.

Encyclopaedia Britannica Company, Merriam-Webster. 2013. Available at: http://www.merriam-webster.com/dictionary/ethics. Accessed February 14, 2013.

Franceschini N, MacCluer JW, Rose KM, et al. 2008. Genome-wide linkage analysis of pulse pressure in American Indians: the Strong Heart Study. *Am J Hypertens.* 21(2):194–199.

Gachupin FC. 2012. Protections to consider when engaging American Indians/Alaska Natives in human subjects research. In Joe JR, Gachupin FC, editors. *Health Soc Iss Native Am Women.* Santa Barbara, CA: Praeger Publishers.

Harmon A. 2010a. Havasupai Case Highlights Risks in DNA Research. *The New York Times.* April 21, 2010. Available at: http://www.nytimes.com/2010/04/22/us/22dnaside. html. Accessed March 2, 2013.

Harmon A. 2010b. Indian Tribe Wins Fight to Limit Research of Its DNA. *The New York Times.* April 21, 2010. Available at: http://www.nytimes.com/2010/04/22/us/ 22dna.html. Accessed March 2, 2013.

Health Research Council of New Zealand. 2010. *Guidelines for Researchers on Health Research Involving Māori.* Available at: http://www.hrc.govt.nz/sites/default/files/

Guidelines%20for%20HR%20on%20Maori-%20Jul10%20revised%20for%20Te%20Ara %20Tika%20v2%20FINAL%5B1%5D.pdf. Accessed March 7, 2013.

Kochanek KD, Xu J, Murphy SL, et al. 2011. Deaths: final data for 2009. *Nat Vit Stat Rep.* 60(3):1–117.

McInnes RR. 2011. 2010 presidential address: culture-the silent language geneticists must learn-genetic research with Indigenous populations. *Am J Human Genetics.* 88:254–261.

National Congress of American Indians, American Indian & Alaska Native Genetics Resource Center. 2013. *Genetics Research and American Indian and Alaska Native Communities.* Available at: http://genetics.ncai.org. Accessed March 7, 2013.

National Congress of State Legislatures. 2009. *Genetic Privacy Laws.* Available at: http:// www.ncsl.org/issues-research/health/genetic-privacy-laws.aspx. Accessed March 6, 2013.

National Heart, Lung, and Blood Institute. 2006. *Strong Heart Family Study.* Available at: http://strongheart.ouhsc.edu/SHFS.pdf. Accessed March 3, 2013.

National Heart, Lung, and Blood Institute. 2013. *Strong Heart Study.* Available at: http://strongheart.ouhsc.edu. Accessed March 3, 2013.

Norris T, Vines PL, Hoeffel EM. 2012. *The American Indian and Alaska Native Population 2010, 2010 Census Briefs.* US Department of Commerce, Economics, and Statistics Administration, US Census Bureau. Available at: http://www.census.gov/prod/ cen2010/briefs/c2010br-10.pdf. Accessed February 21, 2013.

North KE, Almasy L, Goring HH, et al. 2005. Linkage analysis of factors underlying insulin resistance: Strong Heart Family Study. *Obes Res.* 13(11):1877–84.

Office of the High Commissioner for Human Rights, United Nations Human Rights. 2007. *Working Group on the Draft Declaration on the Rights of Indigenous Peoples.* Available at: http://www.ohchr.org/EN/Issues/IPeoples/Pages/WGDraftDeclaration. aspx. Accessed March 7, 2013.

Romero FC, Kanade S. 2000. *Guidelines for Researchers.* Portland, OR: Northwest Portland Area Indian Health Board.

Schiller JS, Lucas JW, Ward BW, et al. 2012. Summary health statistics for US adults: National Health Interview Survey, 2010. *Nat Vital Health Stat.* 10(252).

Spector-Bagdady K. February 12, 2013. "What about Privacy and Progress in Whole Genome Sequencing." Genetic Alliance. Available at: http://www.youtube.com/watch?v=C0P9IlnsJt4&feature=youtu.be. Accessed September 11, 2013.

Tierney P. 2002. *Darkness in El Dorado*. New York, NY: Norton, W.W. & Company, Inc.

US Department of Health and Human Services. 2003. *Summary of the HIPAA Privacy Rule*. Available at: http://www.hhs.gov/ocr/privacy/hipaa/understanding/summary/index.html. Accessed March 6, 2013.

US Department of Health and Human Services. 2009. *HITECH Act Enforcement Interim Final Rule*. Available at: http://www.hhs.gov/ocr/privacy/hipaa/administrative/enforcementrule/hitechenforcementifr.html. Accessed March 6, 2013.

US Department of Health and Human Services. 2013. *The Presidential Commission for the Study of Bioethical Issues*. Available at: http://bioethics.gov/cms/about. Accessed February 12, 2013.

US Department of Health and Human Services, Food and Drug Administration; Center for Devices and Radiological Health; Center for Biologics Evaluation and Research. 2006. *Informed Consent for In Vitro Diagnostic Device Studies Using Leftover Human Specimens that are Not Individually Identifiable: Guidance for Sponsors, Institutional Review Boards, Clinical Investigators and FDA Staff*. Available at: http://www.fda.gov/RegulatoryInformation/Guidances/ucm127022.htm. Accessed March 6, 2013.

US Department of Health and Human Services, Indian Health Service, Division of Program Statistics. 2008. *Regional Differences in Indian Health 2002–2003*. Available at: http://www.ihs.gov/IHS_stats/index.cfm?module=hqPubRD03. Accessed March 3, 2013.

US Department of Health and Human Services, Indian Health Service, Research Program. 2012. *Human Research Participant Protection in the Indian Health Service*. Available at: http://www.ihs.gov/Research/index.cfm. Accessed March 2, 2013.

US Department of Health and Human Services, National Institutes of Health, National Cancer Institute, Office of Biorepositories and Biospecimen Research. 2007. *NCI Best Practices for Biospecimen Resources*. Available at: http://biospecimens.cancer.gov/bestpractices/2011-NCIBestPractices.pdf. Accessed March 6, 2013.

US Department of Health and Human Services, Office for Human Research Protections. 2009. *Code of Federal Regulations, Title 45, Public Welfare, Department of Health and Human Services, Part 46, Protection of Human Subjects.* Available at: http://www.hhs.gov/ohrp/humansubjects/guidance/45cfr46.html. Accessed July 12, 2011.

US Department of Health and Human Services, Office for Human Research Protections. 2011. *ANPRM for Revision to Common Rule: HHS Announces Proposal to Improve Rules Protecting Human Research Subjects.* Available at: http://www.hhs.gov/ohrp/humansubjects/anprm2011page.html. Accessed March 7, 2013.

US Department of Health and Human Services, Office of the Secretary, National Archives and Records Administration, 2013. 45 CFR parts 160 and 164, modifications to the HIPAA privacy, security, enforcement, and breach notification rules under the Health Information Technology for Economic and Clinical Health Act and the Genetic Information Nondiscrimination Act; other modifications to the HIPAA rules; final rule. *Federal Register.* 78(17):5566–5702. Available at: http://www.gpo.gov/fdsys/pkg/FR-2013-01-25/pdf/2013-01073.pdf Accessed March 6, 2013.

US Department of Health and Human Services, US Food and Drug Administration. 2012. *CRF – Code of Federal Regulations Title 21.* Available at: http://www.accessdata.fda.gov/scripts/cdrh/cfdocs/cfcfr/CFRSearch.cfm?CFRPart=50. Accessed July 21, 2013.

US Equal Employment Opportunity Commission. 2009. *Genetic Information Discrimination.* Available at: http://www.eeoc.gov/laws/types/genetic.cfm. Accessed March 6, 2013.

University of New Mexico, Biohazard Compliance for Research. 2013. *Biohazard Compliance Office.* 2013. Available at: http://hsc.unm.edu/som/biohazard. Accessed March 7, 2013.

Wiwchar D. 2004. Nuu-Chah-Nulth Blood Returns to West Coast. *Ha-Shilth-Sa.* 31(25). Available at: http://caj.ca/wp-content/uploads/2010/mediamag/awards2005/(David%20Wiwchar,%20Sept.%2012,%202005)Blood2.pdf. Accessed March 2, 2013.

Wiwchar D. (nd). Nuu-Chah-Nulth Blood Returns to West Coast. *Canadian Assoc Journalists.* Available at: http://caj.ca/wp-content/uploads/2010/mediamag/awards2005/Pages/Community%20Newspaper.htm. Accessed March 2, 2013.

# 12

## Summary: Research in Balance

Teshia G. Arambula Solomon, PhD

### INTRODUCTION

As discussed throughout this book, many Native people and tribes have good reason to distrust researchers as a result of a long, well-documented history of unethical and culturally inappropriate practices imposed upon them. After learning about the lawsuit the Havasupai filed against Arizona State University. Many tribes, particularly in the Southwest, placed moratoriums on research, in some cases even pulling out of ongoing projects. Some have resumed their research activities; others are waiting until they can put protections in place by developing their own research review processes.

While a complete halt to research may prevent cultural violations, it also prevents Native American communities from much needed information and data on population health. As was discussed in Chapter 2, gathering accurate and complete data on Native populations is challenging; however, to have no information leaves leadership empty-handed, without the evidence required to advocate for resources to benefit Native people. To have no data leaves the population virtually invisible. Therefore, as in all things, balance is required. In summary of all that was discussed in the book, in this chapter the benefits of research are discussed and a call to action is suggested to find ways to walk in balance where health research is concerned.

### RESEARCH AS CEREMONY

In *Research is Ceremony*, Wilson describes his experience as an Indigenous researcher by explaining the components of an Indigenous research paradigm and relating the experience of research to the experience of Indigenous ceremony (2008). One purpose of his book is to advocate for a Indigenous research paradigm, and while Wilson finds fault with a Western paradigm of research, he also finds beauty in research, the art of discovery. Indigenous people are taught to have a respect for all things. Scientific discovery in its purest state is the understanding that we do not have the answers; thus, researchers have a healthy respect for what is unknown. There is also great respect for the act of listening and learning. Researchers are compelled to ask questions, discover, and unravel the great mysteries of life. This is done with reverence as ceremony is done with reverence. It also is done with respect, as is ceremony. Traditional ceremony requires preparation on the day of the event and years of training for the ceremonial leader or healer. The same is true of research: it must be properly designed with appropriate controls and methods; the training of a researcher is long and arduous and requires a strong belief in the ideas, the methods, and science. In research, as in ceremony, there are important roles for the participant, without which healing cannot occur. Research also requires storytelling. In the proposal process the researcher explains the problem, what will happen to address the problem or explore it, which participants are involved in the process, what past experience there has been in the line of inquiry, and what the potential outcome might be. After the study is conducted, the researcher looks at the story told by the data. Did the original script unfold exactly as discussed in the proposal or was there an interesting plot twist? Finally, as the story of the research project unfolds the investigator publishes articles and reports that describe the experience in great detail so that others can learn from it.

Ceremony and Indigenous life are all about relationships. Research is about relationships as well; the goal in health research is to understand the relationships that bring people to their best lives. Statistics is the science of understanding relationships between things and using numbers to describe them. Numbers themselves have no meaning until we give them meaning and value. They are simply used in an effort to describe relationships among ideas, behaviors, chemicals, animals, or people. And at the end of the research, as at the end of a ceremony, we hope to have done something to improve life.

## BENEFITS OF RESEARCH

There is no question that atrocities have been committed in the name of research and that many scientists have gone on to fame and fortune at the expense of others, but we must also consider the benefits of research. This author was walking across the campus one day and was struck by the magic of science, technology, and research while watching an older man get into his expensive convertible. At first it was the car that was the focus of attention, but then the man. He was wearing bicycle-racing gear and clearly was in town for a 100-mile charity bike race. Both of his legs were prosthetics. They looked like something out of the latest sci-fi thriller, a flashback to the "Borg" of Star Trek fame: a part-human, part-robot species. It is amazing that technology and science created the opportunity for this man to be able to ride 100 miles just like the other bikers, despite lacking the single most important thing needed to ride a bike—legs. The science that crafted prosthetic limbs capable of sustaining the stress put upon them through long-distance biking is awesome. Researchers did this; they gave this man the opportunity to live a full, self-sufficient life.

Indigenous people were the first scientists, making a scientific and technological impact in fields like medicine, agronomy, pharmacology, and navigation (Weatherford 1988, 1991). Native American (NA) persons developed thousands of varieties of foods including grain, squash, peppers, corn, pumpkin, and beans; discerned uses for rubber and platinum; and managed salmon production (Weatherford 1988, 1991; Pinkerton 1989). NA healers were the first to use medicine including quinine, aspirin, and ipecac (Weatherford 1988, 1991). This important history of Native science is evidence that Native communities have always conducted and benefited from research. They must continue to participate in discoveries that not only sustain humanity but improve lives in ways that are creative, innovative, and otherwise unimaginable.

## CALL TO ACTION

It is imperative that Native communities become intimately involved in the industry of contemporary research. We must train and grow Native scientists to work with Native communities. We must elevate Native needs on the research agenda and on the community agenda. We must elevate Native methods of inquiry to be appreciated as an equal to Western modern methods of science by modifying existing methods and theories and also by creating those that meet the unique needs of our communities.

## Training Native Researchers

There is no single source of information that can accurately describe the scientific and research workforce, particularly in relation to Native Americans, but the belief is that by providing appropriate training in basic research concepts, tools, and methodologies, NA scientists would encourage interest in conducting research in major issues that influence health disparities in Native communities. Unfortunately, a history of unethical research practices and culturally incompetent interpretation of findings, along with little evidence of change in health status among Native people, have created an environment of distrust of research and researchers. Two approaches that have shown to be acceptable to Native communities are (1) using community-based research methods of shared power and decision-making and (2) involving Native researchers as lead investigators and cultural brokers. By increasing the number of Native people involved in health-related research, we can have an impact on the quality of research being conducted and on the scientific knowledge gaps among this underserved population.

## Disparities in Educational Attainment

It is expected that training NA researchers can bring attention and focus to the issues that prevail in the population, thereby reducing health disparities. However, the number of Native students preparing for degrees in the health sciences is very limited. The number of NA scientists and health scientists is significantly lower than any other racial or ethnic group as well as the relative proportion expected based on national population rates (National Science Foundation 2008). We know that this disparity exists along the entire educational pipeline with fewer NA students graduating from high school and college and with fewer applying to graduate programs and health professions programs. Typical barriers to education for any population include poverty and a lack of role models. Approximately 25.7% of NA live below the national poverty level, compared with 12.4% of the total population (US Census Bureau 2011). American Indians report a substantially lower median family income than the population as a whole: $35,700 for American Indian and Alaska Native (AIAN) persons compared with $52,400 for the general population (Kurzweil 2009, US Census Bureau 2004).

According to the US Census, only 13% of AIAN persons aged 25 years and older hold a bachelor's degree or higher compared with the overall population at 28% (National Science Foundation 2008). Recent computations reported in a Harvard Civil Rights project study found that only 51.1% of AIAN 9th graders complete 12th grade with a regular diploma (compared with 75% of Whites, 53.2% of Hispanics, and 50.2% of Blacks). Unlike other groups, the gender gap in high school completion is less than 10 percentage points, with 51% of AIAN girls graduating compared with 48% of boys (Orfield et al. 2004).

The historical separation and isolation of AIAN families and communities from their children in the name of education and the abuse suffered in boarding schools is a shadow that lingers over education in AIAN communities. Although research has shown the health and economic benefits of higher education, barriers remain, particularly among older people. According to Ogbu (1983), minority status is determined by power relationships that subordinate the minority group under a dominant group. Real or perceived continuous long-term discrimination can lead to the development of a hostile or defensive identity that presents itself in direct opposition to the majority values (Simard 1990). Therefore, if schools are for Whites, they are not for Indians. To elders, school usually meant a bad Bureau of Indian Affairs boarding school experience and their memories of school are of people trying to make them forget they were Indian, trying to make them turn against their parents, and telling them that Indian ways were evil (Fedullo 1992). This history has come to create a population that is wary of academic education and research in particular.

Key elements to success in education and training of AIAN persons include providing research training opportunities, professional skills development, peer networks, and role models (Pewardy 1999). Several studies have found the cohort model to be successful in education for AIAN persons and note that peer relationships can be "the single most potent source of influence" (Astin 1993, Nora 1987, Spady 1970, Terenzinin and Pascarella 1997). Jackson et al. (2003) interviewed 15 successful NA college students who grew up on reservations and identified structured social support, faculty and staff warmth, and exposure to college and vocations as key components to success and relevant to mentoring and programmatic support.

Like other underserved students, many AIAN students, particularly those who come from remote or particularly impoverished communities, are less prepared than their non-Native counterparts in math and science and lack writing skills, specifically with regards to language and grammar. Such a deficit puts them at a disadvantage in competing for highly prized internships, scholarships, and other opportunities necessary to becoming a scientist or researcher.

When a student is unable to succeed in the rigorous and competitive environment at a top-tier research institution (particularly a student who has excelled at high school or a smaller college), the student starts to experience self-doubt and begins to question his or her abilities. Often the family and community, as well as the student, have sacrificed so that the student can attend college, taking on financial debt and added responsibility at home. This creates the burden of high expectations for the student. Nearly one-half (between 45–54%) of all Native American students who begin college fail to graduate.

While stronger research is required to validate the experiences of NA students, many activities have been discovered that facilitate persistence and progression in academia for NA trainees. Providing a cohort of Native peers and role models can provide an opportunity for students to take minimal risk in problem solving and not lose face by asking questions. The cohort also provides the sense of community that students miss when away from family and appreciates the students' unique cultural practices or customs, a support unavailable in a fraternity or sorority or other college group. Training students to pursue the long and arduous career in the sciences requires role models and catalysts—people who can spark interest, facilitate resources, and serve as champions. Research indicates that support, guidance, and role modeling are key functions of the mentoring relationship (Grossman and Rhodes 2002, Kram 1985). The literature on mentoring is divided regarding who makes the best mentor, with some studies showing that cross-race relationships can be effective for minority students, while other studies indicating they may be less effective (Moses 1989, Pounds 1987, Rowe 1989, Hughes 1988). For Native students, however, the limited number of Native investigators available to serve as role models complicates the problem. In 2011 there were 22 AIAN faculty on the University of Arizona main and health science campuses, and 10 of those were tenured faculty (<1% of the total). One way this limitation has been overcome at the Native American Research and Training Center (NARTC) is to provide opportunities for undergraduates to study under graduate students and post-doctorates and for graduate students and post-doctorates to learn from and work with junior faculty from around the country. NARTC also partners with Native organizations around the country to encourage Native-focused scientific conferences and give students the opportunity to shine at such conferences and meetings, so they may receive recognition from community leaders.

Academic support in the form of tutoring in math, science, writing and taking entrance exams for health professions schools or graduate school helps students compete with less disadvantaged students. This is provided in the form of advice, direct assistance, group tutoring, and financial support.

Providing flexibility that allows students to participate in essential cultural and community activities helps them achieve their goals in a less-stressful environment. It is important to set clear expectations of what is needed to achieve their academic goals and to work with them to determine how to respond to competing activities, manage workloads and schedules, and negotiate with parents on their expectations.

Helping students manage the expectations of family members and themselves is important. Sharing stories of a mentor's struggles and overcoming those hardships is an effective vicarious learning tool. Counseling with honesty, clarity, and empathy will assist students in finding pathways that meet their career goals rather than abandoning dreams because there is an academic bad fit. Exposing students to a range of career options allows them to explore the possibilities and find a better fit for themselves. By preparing a critical mass of Native investigators in health, Native communities can assume a leadership role in research agenda setting and in the development of the research industry. Native scientists who can successfully navigate the research and academic worlds and the Native community can be facilitators for the elimination of health disparities and for scientific inquiry.

## Elevate Native Health on the Research Agenda and on the Community Agenda

The Canadian Institutes of Health Research developed a national research protocol and process when working with the Aboriginal peoples of Canada and established an Institute of Aboriginal People's Health in 2000, whose mission is to lead the research agenda for Aboriginal health. The US Department of Health and Human Services has a tribal consultation process and follows the guidelines of institutional review boards (IRBs) certified by the federal Assurance for the Protection of Human Subjects. The Indian Health Service (IHS) houses an IRB for studies conducted in their facilities, and tribes are increasingly creating their own IRBs or other human participants protection protocol. A national research protocol, like that of the CIHR with the development of research principles specific to Native communities that expands upon the basic human participants protection requirements and the dissemination of this information, would benefit the tribal and scientific communities. In her book, *Indigenous Storywork*, Archibald (2008) suggests and explains seven research principles: (1) respect, (2) responsibility, (3) reciprocity, (4) reverence, (5) holism, (6) interrelatedness, and (7) synergy. These principles are relevant to research with all peoples, but given the unique political relationship between the United States and NA tribes, they are particularly important to Native people.

In addition to protecting human participants in Native research, honesty in proposing, performing, and reporting research is also important, particularly when Native students are involved. Native investigators put their reputations in the community at risk when they conduct research, and while a non-Native investigator can leave a community should there be issues, a Native investigator will be held to a higher standard. Failure to keep promises has repercussions related to trust. Researchers need to accurately represent student and community member contributions to research proposals, papers, and reports.

### Respect Native Methods of Knowing and Scientific Inquiry

As mentioned above, Native people are natural scientists. The ancient Pima were originators of complex irrigation systems, transforming arid desert land into gardens of wheat, beans, squash, and the much-desired Pima cotton. For generations the Pima have participated in studies on diabetes, contributing to the body of science on diabetes risk and management through the gift of participation in many research studies. Today, Alaska Natives teach math and science to state and national standards using ancient teachings of sustainable life including salmon harvesting and star navigation (Adams and Lipka 2003).

It is in this spirit that Native researchers call for the development of an Indigenous research paradigm for the 21st century, which discovers solutions to problems that plague Native communities, commands respect for the people and their cultures, and uses methods that honor the ancient ways of knowing that have endured over generations. An Indigenous paradigm is needed to ensure the cultural relevance of research strategies and to provide effective, sustainable, lifelong lessons. As previously mentioned, community-based participatory research methods have been found not only to be acceptable research methods in Native communities but also to be insisted upon in many Native communities as methods that incorporate the respect for Native sovereignty. Other research methods have also been found to be approaches that fit well with Native ways of knowing, including talking circles. Theoretical methods like the Social Ecological Model offer a context compatible with an Indigenous paradigm (McLeroy et al. 1988). This model requires approaching behavioral change, assessment, and analysis by looking at the whole rather than by breaking things down into individual component parts, a western approach. It uses the whole as a laboratory, looking at all possible influences and avenues of intervention as opposed to the isolation and creation of an unnatural environment through the control of variables. Most Indigenous people look at the world through relationships; people are introduced by their clanship, their relationship to their family, and perhaps the community to whom they are speaking. One research methodology currently in the spotlight due to the development of Facebook and other popular social media is social network analysis (Wasserman and Faust 1999). This method of organizing and understanding the world is all about relationships and the power of influence. It has been used for sociology, business, and mathematics to a greater degree than for public health but is becoming increasingly popular (Luke and Harris 2007). Native ways of knowing could well inform further development and application of this methodology to understand patterns of health and disease. Another research strategy that is very popular among Native communities in the United States is digital storytelling. The title itself attracts Native people, for whom oral communication has been the primary form of transmission of important information for generations.

While these forms of research (and others) must be further developed in order to meet the needs of Native communities, there is also a need to develop innovative strategies, particularly in data collection and analysis. In the United

States, Native communities are often left out of large, national studies or at least omitted from analysis, with the explanation that the Native American population is too small for significant findings in statistical analysis. It is worth repeating that a lack of information creates invisible populations and inaccurate or incomplete descriptions of health concerns. Such was the case with cancer data at the national level until an innovative team developed by the Centers for Disease Control and IHS began to create a data linkage methodology at a regional level (Espey et al. 2008). These analytical methods provided a picture of the wide variation in cancer disparities across AIAN regions in the United States, indicating distinct needs based on variations in risk. Such methods are now being studied in Indigenous communities around the world.

Rutman and others have utilized multiyear analysis methods to create sufficient sample sizes for analysis when reviewing and reporting behavioral risk factor surveillance data (Rutman et al. 2008; Rohde et al. 2013; Chou et al. 2013). Despite these creative methods, a full picture of both the health status of all Native Americans and information for individual Native communities is incomplete. Further research and development of methods of analysis would greatly benefit distinct communities in the delivery of healthcare, health promotion, and disease prevention.

One resource that has been effective in increasing the amount and quality of public health research in the United States are the tribal epidemiology centers (TECs). The IHS Division of Epidemiology established the first TEC in 1997 to serve AIAN tribal and urban communities by managing public health information systems, investigating diseases of concern, managing disease prevention and control programs, responding to public health emergencies, and coordinating with state and national public health authorities.

## SUMMARY

By fully participating as leaders in the research enterprise, Native people possess the voice and power to advocate for Native communities. In this book we demonstrate the power of Native investigators as authors and researchers. The emphasis is placed on respectful and ethically sound research; in addition, Native communities must invest in the education and training of children in science and math as well as in traditional practices in order for them to address the key issues in communities as Native scientists. Native health must be elevated on the national, state, local, and tribal research agendas. Methods of science and discovery that meet the unique issues and concerns of Native communities must be addressed. The sovereignty of Native nations must be sacrosanct and rights and privileges must be protected. With a fully developed research program, health standards of Native people will be raised to be equivalent to or better than those of the non-Native communities within which they live. In speaking about the need for an Indigenous research paradigm, Wilson (2008) emphasizes that through research,

> we can provide ways to celebrate the uniqueness and glory of Indigenous cultures, while allowing for the critical examination of shortcomings. It will encourage a greater appreciation of Indigenous history and worldviews, thus allowing Indigenous peoples to look towards the future while neither demonizing nor romanticizing the past.

By putting research in balance, Native American researchers can accomplish the same.

## REFERENCES

Archibald J. 2008. *Indigenous Storywork: Educating the Heart, Mind, Body, and Spirit.* Vancouver, BC: UBC Press.

Astin AW. 1993. *What Matters in College? Four Critical Years Revisited.* San Francisco, CA: Jossey-Bass.

Chou CF, Sherrod C, Zhang X, et al. 2013. Barriers to eye care among people aged 40 years and older with diagnosed diabetes, 2006–2010. *Diabetes Care.* [Epub ahead of print.] Available at: http://www.ncbi.nlm.nih.gov/pubmed/24009300. Accessed September 11, 2013.

Espey DK, Wiggins CL, Jim MA, et al. 2008. Methods for improving cancer surveillance data in American Indian and Alaska Native populations. *Cancer.* 113(5 suppl):1120–1130.

Fedullo M. 1992. *Light of the Feather: Pathways Through Contemporary Indian America.* New York, NY: William Morrow.

Grossman JB, Rhodes JE. 2002. The test of time: predictors and effects of duration in youth mentoring relationships. *Am J Community Psychol.* 30(2):199–219.

Hughes MS. 1988. Developing leadership potential for minority women. In: Sagaria MAD, editor. *Empowering Women: Leadership Development Strategies on Campus (New Directions for Student Services).* San Francisco, CA: Jossey-Bass. p. 63–75.

Jackson AP, Smith SA, Hill CL. 2003. Academic persistence among Native American college students. *J College Student Dev.* 44(4):548–565.

Kawagley A, Norris-Tull D. 1995. Incorporation of the worldviews of indigenous cultures: A dilemma in the practice and teaching of western science. Paper presented at: Third International History, Philosophy, and Science Teaching Conference, Minneapolis, MN: October 29–November 2, 1995.

Kram KE. 1985. *Mentoring at Work: Developmental Relationships in Organizational Life.* Glenview, IL: Scott Foresman.

Kurzweil J, Hundt LM. 2007. Meaningful mentoring – Native American and Latino success stories. *SACNAS News.* Available at: http://sciencecareers.sciencemag.org/ career_magazine/previous_issues/articles/2007_10_05/science.opms.r0700041. Accessed July 21, 2013.

Luke DA, Harris JK. 2007. Network analysis in public health: History, methods, and applications. *Annu Rev Public Health.* 28:69–93.

McLeroy K, Bibeau D, Steckler A, et al. 1988. An ecological perspective on health promotion programs. *Health Educ Quarterly.* 15(4):351–377.

Moses YT. Black women in academe: issues and strategies. Paper presented at: Conference of the Association of American Colleges, Washington, DC, August 1989. ERIC Document Reproduction Services No. ED 311-817. Available at: http://files.eric. ed.gov.ezproxy1.library.arizona.edu/fulltext/ED311817.pdf. Accessed September 11, 2013.

National Science Foundation, Division of Science Resources Statistics. 2008. *Graduate Students and Postdoctorates in Science and Engineering: Fall 2006. Detailed Statistical Tables/NSF 08-306.* Available at: http://www.nsf.gov/statistics/nsf08306. Accessed July 21, 2013.

Nora A. 1987. Determinants of retention among Chicano college students: a structural model. *Res Higher Educ.* 26:31–39.

Ogbu JU. 1983. Minority status and schooling in plural societies. *Comp Educ Rev.* 17(2):169–190.

Orfield G, Losen D, Wald J, et al. 2004. *Losing Our Future: How Minority Youth are Being Left Behind by the Graduation Rate Crisis.* Cambridge, MA: The Civil Rights Project at Harvard University.

Pewardy C. 1999. *The Holistic Medicine Wheel: An Indigenous Model of Teaching and Learning. Winds of Change 28–30.* Available at: http://www.library.wisc.edu/edvrc/docs/public/pdfs/SEEDReadings/HolisticMedicineWheel.pdf. Accessed July 21, 2013.

Pinkerton E, editor. 1989. *Co-Operative Management of Local Fisheries: New Directions for Improved Management and Community Development.* Vancouver, BC: University of British Columbia Press.

Pounds AW. 1987. Black students' needs on predominantly White campuses. In: Wright DJ, editor. *Responding to the Needs of Today's Minority Students.* Hoboken, NJ: Wiley Sons and Incorporated.

Rowe MP. 1989. What actually works? The one-to-one approach. In: Pearson CS, Shavlik DL, Touchton JG, editors. *Educating the Majority: Women Challenge Tradition in Higher Education.* New York, NY: American Council on Education and Macmillan. p. 375–384.

Rohde K, Boles M, Bushore CJ, et al. 2013. Smoking-related knowledge, attitudes, and behaviors among Alaska Native people: a population-based study. *Int J Circumpolar Health.* Aug 5;72.

Rutman S, Park A, Castor M, et al. 2008. Urban American Indian and Alaska native youth: Youth Risk Behavior Survey 1997–2003. *Matern Child Health J.* 12:S76–S81.

Simard J-J. 1990. White ghosts, red shadows: the reduction of North American Indians. In: Clifton JA, editor. *The Invented Indian: Cultural Fictions and Government Policies.* New Brunswick, NJ: Transaction Publishers. p. 333–369.

Snively G, Corsiglia J. 2000. *Discovering Indigenous Science: Implications for Science Education.* Available at: http://citeseerx.ist.psu.edu/viewdoc/download?doi=10.1.1.123.2213&rep=rep1&type=pdf. Accessed July 21, 2013.

Spady W. 1970. Dropouts from higher education: an interdisciplinary review and synthesis. *Interchange.* 1(1):64–85.

Terenzini PT, Pascarella ET. 1977. Voluntary freshman attrition and patterns of social and academic integration in a university: A test of a conceptual model. *Res Higher Educ.* 6:25–43.

US Census Bureau. 2004. *We the People: American Indians and Alaska Natives in the United States. Census 2000 Special Reports.* Available at: http://www.census.gov/prod/2006pubs/censr-28.pdf. Accessed July 21, 2013.

US Census Bureau. 2012. *The American Indian and Alaska Native Population: 2010.* Available at: http://www.census.gov/prod/cen2010/briefs/c2010br-10.pdf. Accessed July 21, 2013.

Wasserman S, Faust K. 1999. *Social Networks Analysis: Methods and Applications.* Cambridge, MA: Cambridge University Press.

Wilson S. 2008. *Research is Ceremony: Indigenous Research Methods.* Black Point, Nova Scotia: Fernwood Publishing.

Weatherford J. 1988. *Indian Givers: How the Indians of the Americas Transformed the World.* Toronto, ON: Random House.

Weatherford J. 1991. *Native Roots: How the Indians Enriched America.* Toronto, ON: Random House.

# Contributors

## EDITORS

**Teshia G. Arambula Solomon, PhD,** is a member of the Choctaw Nation. She is the great granddaughter of Lila and Forbes Manning, original enrollees of the Choctaw Nation, the granddaughter of Vera Manning and Buel Braudrick, and the daughter of Jeraldine Braudrick. Her patrilineal heritage is as granddaughter of Rosa and Trinidad Arambula of Durango, Mexico, and the daughter of Louis Arambula. Dr. Solomon has over 20 years of experience in health, education, and research projects with Native American and Latino populations. She is the director of the Native American Research and Training Center (NARTC), a regents-appointed institution to provide support and technical assistance to the Native American communities in Arizona. She is an associate professor in the Department of Family and Community Medicine at the University of Arizona. She currently is the principal investigator of the Research and Training Cores for the American Indian Research Centers for Health, a collaboration with the Inter-Tribal Council of Arizona. She is also a co-principal investigator with the Partnership for Native American Cancer Prevention, University of Arizona Cancer Center and Northern Arizona University, responsible for the community outreach program. Dr. Solomon's research focuses on cancer prevention and control, Indigenous health and science workforce development, and maternal and child health. Dr. Solomon mentors Native American undergraduate and graduate students, community members, and junior faculty pursuing careers in the health sciences. She is a founding member of the Native Research Network, Inc., and has served as co-chair, secretary-treasurer, and treasurer of the nonprofit group and holds membership in several groups, including the International Group on Indigenous Health Measurement and the Advisory Board for the Mayo

Clinic Spirit of EAGLES program. She holds an appointment with the National Cancer Institute as senior research advisor to assess and further develop opportunities for career development for Indigenous researchers. Dr. Solomon has served as an advocate for social justice in the health and well-being of disenfranchised populations through her research, teaching, and service to the community, particularly to benefit Indigenous people, particularly women and children.

**Leslie L. Randall, RN, MPH, BSN,** is a member of the NiMiiPu Nation, a Nez Perce Tribal member, and is the daughter of Vernon Edward Waters, son of Samuel Watters and Blanche Hung, and Mazie Margaret Moses, daughter of Lillian and Elias Moses. She is a direct descendant of War Chief Ollicut, younger brother of Chief Joseph of the Wallowa Band of Nez Perce. She attended Oregon Health Sciences University and the School of Public Health, University of Hawai'i at Mānoa, and has worked in Maternal Child Health (MCH) for the past 22 years. Ms. Randall currently sits as a member of Nez Perce Tribal Employment Rights Commission, the Healthy Native Babies Project Advisory Group, the Nimiipu Health Board, and the Washington State University Native American Health Science Advisory Committee. She is a standing member of the Agency for Health Care Quality and Research/HQER study committee and a past member of the Nez Perce Enterprise Board, and is a private consultant. Ms. Randall is also a former co-chair and a founding member of the Native Research Network, Inc. and past chair of the American Indian/Alaska Native/Native Hawaiian Caucus of the American Public Health Association. Ms. Randall has served as an Indian Health Service (IHS) institutional review board (IRB) member since 1994, first at the Aberdeen Area IHS IRB and then at the National IHS IRB. She worked for Indian Health Service from 1992 to 1997 and then for the Centers for Disease Control and Prevention (CDC) from 1997 to 2007. Through a Memorandum of Agreement between IHS and CDC, Ms. Randall worked on reproductive health/behavioral risk surveys and provided technical assistance for the design, implementation, analysis, training and dissemination of findings to tribes. She was the senior MCH epidemiologist first to the National Indian Health Service National Epidemiology Program and then to the Northwest Portland Area Indian Health Board. She has presented on such diverse topics as grief, infant mortality, and race relations to local, regional, national, and international audiences. She met with the New Zealand Conciliator from the Office of Race Relations at his request because of her work on race relations. Ms. Randall currently resides on her homelands on the Nez Perce Reservation where she is completing a doctorate in nursing at Washington State University, a source of pride for the university (see http://nursing.wsu.edu/Media-Dashboard/ News&Media/PhD-scholar-Leslie-Randal-in-the-news.html). Throughout her career, she has been a tireless researcher for and an outspoken advocate of Indian health, particularly for mothers and children, and believes all Native people should have access to quality care. Ms. Randall has worked in support of tribal sovereignty and self-determination throughout her career and believes that sovereignty needs to be guarded and maintained.

## AUTHORS

**Doris M. Cook, PhD, MPH,** is a member of the Akwesasne Mohwak Nation, a former co-chair of the Native Research Network, Inc., and has done extensive work in health policy and developing research ethics protocols for health research projects involving Indigenous peoples. Between 2003 and 2007, she was the manager of Aboriginal Ethics Policy Development in the Ethics Office of the Canadian Institutes of Health Research (CIHR), Canada's premier national health funding agency. In that capacity, she coordinated the development of new Aboriginal research guidelines. The guidelines are intended to promote beneficial research by providing protections for Aboriginal research participants. Prior to her work with CIHR, she spent 10 years in the Policy Division at Health Canada, where she was the lead analyst on files such as ethics, genetics, and assisted human reproduction. She was part of the Canadian delegation that negotiated the United Nations Educational, Scientific, and Cultural Organization's Declaration on the Human Genome and Human Rights and represented Canada at the Council of Europe's Standing Committee on Ethics. She is currently an independent consultant working in the areas of policy development, program and organizational management, program evaluation, public health planning, and research ethics with clients that include a center of excellence in Aboriginal health, a national Aboriginal organization, national government departments, a university involved in the development of a research ethics policy on benefits sharing with Aboriginal communities, and local tribal/band governments. She is also involved in ethics review at the community level in her home community, the Mohawk Territories of Akwesasne.

**William L. Freeman, MD, MPH, CIP,** has served in Indian health his entire medical career. The summer of 1971, following his first year of medical school, he worked for the Swinomish Indian Tribal Community to develop and conduct a health survey of its members, as requested by the tribal chairman. He stayed in contact with many Swinomish people throughout medical school, and both his family medicine clerkship and his family medicine residency community rotation were with the practice in Anacortes, Washington, where most Swinomish people received their health care. After completing his residency and receiving his MPH, he began his career of 25 ½ years in the Indian Health Service (IHS) at the Lummi Indian Tribal Health Center, where he served from 1977 to 1990. From 1990 to 2002, he was director of the IHS Research Program, and chair of the IHS IRB, which supports and encourages community-based participatory research (CBPR) and promotes the ethical conduct of research in AIAN communities. Since his retirement from IHS, Dr. Freeman has served at the Northwest Indian College as the human protections administrator and the program director for the Center for Health. His research includes resiliency and strengths of Native people, CBPR, the ethics of research involving Native communities, understanding the knowledge, attitudes, beliefs, and behaviors about HIV, health services research, and program evaluation. Of particular interest to him is the role of individual and community participants in research, their concerns, and their desires for research. Because he is a living kidney donor, he also has a professional and personal interest in the care of living organ donors before and after donation, and the ethics of living kidney donation. He currently serves on the United Network of Organ Sharing Living Donor Committee. He and his wife, Carolyn Robbins, are privileged to live on the Lummi Reservation alongside the proud Lummi people.

**Francine C. Gachupin, PhD, MPH, CIP,** is a member of the Pueblo of Jemez, New Mexico. Dr. Gachupin has extensive experience working with American Indian tribal communities, focusing primarily on chronic disease surveillance, public health practice, epidemiology, and research. She obtained her doctorate in Anthropology from the University of New Mexico and her Master of Public Health in Epidemiology from the University of Washington in Seattle. Her work has been based primarily at tribal epidemiology centers including northwest, northern plains, and southwest tribes. She has been principal investigator to several projects focused on behavioral risk factors for adults and youth, cancer, dementia, diet and nutrition, domestic violence, eye disease, heart disease mortality, injury prevention, and population genetics. Dr. Gachupin has also worked in human participants protection as an IRB chair, co-chair, committee member; Health and Human Services Secretary's Advisory Committee on Human Research Protections member; and operations manager for the University of New Mexico human research protections office. She is an assistant professor at the University of Arizona, College of Medicine, Department of Family and Community Medicine. She is also the assistant director of the Native American Research and Training Center and assistant director, Arizona Cancer Center, Health Disparities Institute.

**Felicia Schanche Hodge, DrPH,** is a member of the Wailaki Indian tribe from California. Dr. Hodge has over 30 years of experience in Indian health, education, and research projects. She is the founder and director of the Center for American Indian/Indigenous Research & Education, which supports research, evaluation, policy development, education, planning, prevention, and community service activities. She holds a joint faculty appointment in the School of Public Health (Health Services) and the School of Nursing (Primary Care). Dr. Hodge has also served as the chair of the American Indian Studies Interdepartmental Program, and carries a personal interest in cancer prevention and control among American Indians. Dr. Hodge earned an MPH in healthcare (1976) and a DrPH in health administration from the University of California at Berkeley in 1987. Following her master's degree, she worked for 36 reservation tribes in the states of Washington, Oregon, and Idaho, where she headed up and incorporated a tribal advocacy center (Northwest Portland Area Indian Health Board), testifying before Congress for clinic and training needs of tribes. Dr. Hodge's research includes tobacco cessation and control; breast, cervical, and colorectal cancer screening; Type II diabetes; nutrition; wellness; and cancer symptom management, including pain and depression. She has employed the use of "talking circles" and storytelling in her research protocols since the early 1990s, with strong outcomes in changing perceptions, knowledge, and improved health-related behaviors. She completed a four-year appointment to the National Institute of Nursing Research's National Advisory Council and is currently a member of the Agency for Healthcare Research and Quality women's expert group. Dr. Hodge teaches Research Methods among

Indigenous Populations for the American Indian Studies program and California Indian History for the History Department. In the School of Nursing, she teaches two doctoral seminars as well as classes in Responsible Conduct of Research and Family Nursing Theory.

**Jennie R. Joe, PhD, MPH,** is a member of the Navajo Nation and retired professor in the Department of Family and Community Medicine and former director of the Native American Research and Training Center in the College of Medicine at the University of Arizona. She also held a faculty appointment in the Department of American Indian Studies at the university. Some of her research activities have included American Indian children and youth with type II diabetes; breast and cervical cancer screening; culturally based substance abuse treatment programs; traditional tribal medicine, disability and rehabilitation; and the impact of health disparities on American Indians and Alaska Natives. Professor Joe has served on a number of national and international organizations, including the Institute of Medicine, the Advisory Council for the National Heart, Lung, and Blood Institute as well as the Institute of Aboriginal People's Health, an institute within CIHR. As a researcher, she continues to be involved with a number of health-related studies that are conducted in partnership with tribal groups throughout the country. As an educator and a mentor, she continues to work with students from multicultural backgrounds.

**Lillian Tom-Orme, RN, PhD, MPH, FAAN,** a member of the Navajo Nation, was born and raised on the Navajo Indian reservation in New Mexico. Dine' was her first language and she remains fluent in her native tongue. Dr. Tom-Orme is a research assistant professor in the Department of Internal Medicine, University of Utah School of Medicine, and has adjunct appointments in the Department of Pediatrics and the College of Nursing. Dr. Tom-Orme holds graduate degrees in transcultural nursing and public health from the University of Utah. In addition, she serves as Native American Research Liaison through an inter-agency personnel agreement with the National Cancer Institute. Dr. Tom-Orme has been active in local and national committees including the American Diabetes Association's Awakening the Spirit Program, the American Indian/Alaska Native/Native Hawai'ian Caucus of the American Public Health Association, the National Alaska Native/ American Indian Nurses Association, advisory member of the NIH Center for Health Disparity and Minority Health, panel of experts member to the Office on Women's Health of the Department of Health and Human Services, the Native Research Network, Inc., the Network for Cancer Control Research among American Indian and Alaska Native Populations, the national IHS IRB, the National Coalition of Ethnic Minority Nurses Associations, and as reviewer for the *Journal of American Indian Education*. Dr. Tom-Orme was employed by the Utah Department of Health in tuberculosis control, refugee health, diabetes, and primary care for 15 years. She is a consultant and author in transcultural nursing and public health. Her current research includes patterns of cancer care and chronic health conditions in American Indians and Alaska Natives.

**Joey Quenga, BA,** is of Chamoru descent and is executive director of the TOA Institute. Mr. Quenga oversees all aspects of work at the TOA Institute, a nonprofit organization that helps improve the lives of Pacific Islander people through policy analysis, education, research, programs, and services. Mr. Quenga also directs the Pacific Islander Epidemiology Center, a national program housed at the TOA Institute, which focuses on collecting, analyzing, and reporting on the health status of Pacific Islanders in the United States. In addition to his roles at the TOA Institute, he is the co-director of Kutturan Chamoru Performers, a nonprofit volunteer group dedicated to learning and promoting the traditional folkdance of the Micronesian Marianas Islands. He has been awarded for his community service to the Chamoru community, and received the Tan Chong Padula Humanitarian of the Year Award and Maga'lahi Award for "Off-Island Contribution" Guam Governors Award. He received his BA in Communications from San Francisco State University in 1996.

**Raynald Samoa, MD,** is an assistant professor in the Department of Clinical Diabetes, Endocrinology & Metabolism at City of Hope Hospital in Duarte, California. Dr. Samoa is uniquely trained both as an adult and pediatric endocrinologist. Dr. Samoa did much of his training at University of Southern California, Los Angeles County (USC+LAC), completing a fellowship in endocrinology, diabetes, and metabolism as well as an internship and residency in combined internal medicine and pediatrics. He served as chief resident at USC's Women's & Children's Hospital. Dr. Samoa pursues a variety of clinical research topics in endocrinology, from adrenal disorders in children to studying the effects of obesity on vulnerable populations. He is working on several obesity-intervention projects in Pacific Islander communities locally and abroad. As a member of multiple boards of Native Hawaiian and Pacific Islander Community Based Organizations (CBOs), he has laid the groundwork for many proposed research projects by establishing strong ties with community providers and community-based organizations.

**Delight E. Satter, MPH,** is a member of the Confederated Tribes of Grand Ronde and is associate director for Tribal Support in the Office for State, Tribal, Local and Territorial Support, CDC, where she coordinates CDC programs and policies that benefit or affect American Indian/Alaska Native (AIAN) populations, including CDC's Tribal Consultation Policy and Tribal Advisory Committee. She is the principal advisor and main liaison with policy-level officials, and acts as CDC's principal contact for all AIAN public health activities. Prior to joining CDC, she directed the American Indian Research Program, which she founded in 1998 at the UCLA Center for Health Policy Research (the Center), one of the nation's preeminent policy research centers. Ms. Satter is a strong advocate for the health and well-being of urban and rural/reservation American Indians. Her work at the Center focused on Native cancer, tobacco prevention, and policy opportunities for tribes, epidemiologic profile of Native elders, evaluation of a Native infant health program targeting at risk pregnancies and children, and evaluation and technical assistance on youth mental health care access. She also served as a key staff member on the development of the California Health Interview Survey. She served as board member for the California Pan Ethnic Health Network and Native American Cancer Research; served on the inaugural US Secretary of Health and Human Services Advisory Committee on Minority Health; was a founding member of the Native Research Network Board of Directors and the CDC's American Indian, Alaska Native, and Native Hawaiian Coalition; and is past president of the American Indian, Alaska Native, and Native Hawaiian Caucus of the American Public Health Association. Ms. Satter was a Public Health Prevention Service fellow with CDC, a Morris K. Udall American Indian Congressional Intern to the Honorable Bruce F. Vento (dec.), and an intern at the Minnesota Department of Public Health. She received her master's degree in public health from the University of Minnesota and bachelor's degree in anthropology from the University of Washington.

**Roxanne Struthers, RN, PhD, CHTP, AHN-BC, CTN,** (dec.) was a member of the Red Lake Ojibwe tribe and was born and raised on the White Earth Reservation in northwestern Minnesota. She was a pioneering American

Indian nursing educator, researcher, author, healer, and leader. Dr. Struthers, an assistant professor at the University of Minnesota School of Nursing, was one of a limited number of American Indians to hold a doctorate in nursing (14 at publishing time). At the time of her death, she was president-elect of the National Alaska Native and American Indian Nurses Association (NANAINA) and was serving on the Department of Health and Human Services' National Advisory Council on Nurse Education and Practice. Dr. Struthers earned her doctorate in nursing from the University of Minnesota in 1999 and was a certified healing touch practitioner, holistic nurse, and certified transcultural nurse. She was internationally recognized for her research on Indian health issues, including diabetes, tobacco use, traditional Indian healing, and historical trauma. With her NANAINA colleague, Dr. John Lowe, she published a groundbreaking model for culturally competent Indian nursing practice, as part of the Nursing in Native American Culture project. In addition to devoting her career to improving the health of Indian people, Dr. Struthers worked tirelessly to help other Native nurses gain access to academic and research careers. At the University of Minnesota, she was a key faculty member on the American Indian MS-to-PhD Nursing Science Bridge, a NIH-funded project designed to double the number of Native nurses with doctoral degrees. She was also director of the University of Minnesota's Native Nurses Career Opportunity Program.

**Maile Taualii, PhD, MPH,** is an assistant professor of Health Policy and Management in the Office of Public Health Studies at the University of Hawai'i, Manoa, where she brings cultural, ethical, and community-oriented perspectives to the instruction of public health, and director of the Native Hawaiian Epidemiology Center, Papa Ola Lokahi, and heads the Native Hawaiian and Indigenous Health specialization within the Master's of Public Health program. Dr. Taualii received her PhD in Health Services with an emphasis in public health informatics and public health genetics from the University of Washington, where she also completed her Master's in Public Health. Dr. Taualii is the founding director of the Native Hawaiian Epidemiology Center housed at Papa Ola Lokahi, the Native Hawaiian Health Board. The Native Hawaiian Epidemiology Center performs targeted and coordinated epidemiological investigations and works in partnership with communities, agencies, health officials, and others in crafting strategic interventions to retard or reverse health problems. Prior appointments include serving as the scientific director for the Urban Indian Health Institute, an IHS-designated Tribal Epidemiology Center for nearly 10 years. She is the recipient of a Bioinformatics/Public Health Informatics Fellowship and has expertise in development, evaluation, and utilization of data and data systems. A primary research focus for Dr. Taualii is the utility and validity of health information for racial minorities. She is the past chair of the American Public Health Association, American Indian/Alaska Native/Native Hawaiian Caucus, a board member of the Native Hawaiian and Pacific Islander Health Alliance, vice chair of the International Indigenous Centre for Health Intelligence, and the a past co-chair for the Native Research Network, Inc. In 2007, Dr. Taualii was awarded the Mentors and Community Legacy Award for Women of Color Empowered.

**Thomas K. Welty, MD, MPH**, is a medical epidemiologist and family physician who retired in 1997 from the Public Health Service after 26 years of service with IHS and CDC. He served as the principal investigator of the Strong Heart Study, the Sioux Cancer Study, the Aberdeen Area Infant Mortality Study, and several other studies related to Indian health. Dr. Welty continues to be an advocate for working and consulting with Native communities from inception to conclusion of studies. He has mentored many students and staff throughout the years and continues to provide a working example of how to work with Native communities. Since his retirement, he continues to serve as co-investigator for the Strong Heart Study and has provided voluntary service in tuberculosis control and AIDS prevention in Cameroon, West Africa.

# Index